MATHA J. RUSSELL

DEPRESSION IN WOMEN

Practical Strategies and Mindfulness Practices for Women

Contents

1

Introduction

It was a day like any other or so it seemed. The sun was shining, birds chirping, and the world bustling with life. Yet, for me, the world felt like a dark and desolate place a place devoid of joy, hope, and meaning.

I had always been the strong one the one who held everything together, no matter how turbulent life became. But beneath the facade of strength lay a profound sense of emptiness a gnawing ache that refused to be silenced. Depression crept into my life slowly, insidiously, like a thief in the night. At first, it was just a whisper, a fleeting sense of sadness or unease. But as time went on, the whispers grew louder, more persistent, until they drowned out the sound of everything else.

I tried to ignore it, to push through the pain and pretend like everything was okay. But the more I tried to bury my feelings, the more they consumed me. I felt like I was suffocating, drowning in a sea of darkness with no hope of escape. It wasn't until I hit rock bottom that I realized I couldn't do it alone. I reached out for help with therapy, medication, and support from loved ones. And slowly, ever so, I began to find my way back to the light.

It wasn't easy. There were days when the darkness threatened to engulf me once again, days when I felt like giving up. But with each step forward, I gained strength, courage, and resilience. I learned to embrace my pain, to acknowledge it without letting it define me. Today, I am grateful for the journey I have traveled for the lessons learned, the growth experienced, and the person I have become. Depression will always be a part of my story, but it no longer holds power over me. I am stronger than I ever thought possible, and I know that whatever challenges lie ahead, I will face them with grace, courage, and unwavering hope.

My journey with depression is just one of millions a testament to the silent struggle that so many women face each day. Depression knows no bounds of age, race, or background. It can strike anyone, anywhere, at any time. Yet, despite its prevalence, depression remains shrouded in silence and stigma. Many women suffer in silence, afraid to seek help or share their struggles with others. But the truth is, that depression thrives in darkness. It feeds on isolation and shame, robbing us of our voice and our sense of worth.

That's why I wrote this book to shine a light on the darkness, to break the silence, and to offer hope to those who are struggling. In the pages that follow, we will explore the intricacies of depression in women, the causes, symptoms, and their impact on daily life. We will also delve into practical strategies for managing depression, from self-care and mindfulness to seeking professional help and building a support network.

But more than that, this book is a testament to the resilience of the human spirit to the capacity for healing, growth, and transformation that lies within every one of us.

The Importance of Self-Help for Depression in Women

Depression, a common mental health disorder impacting millions of women worldwide, can seem like an insurmountable impediment to living a successful and happy life. While getting professional support is critical for depression management, the importance of self-help measures cannot be emphasized. Empowering women with the tools and techniques to actively participate in their healing path is not only beneficial but also necessary in confronting the numerous issues of depression. Here are numerous arguments that emphasize the necessity of self-help for depression in women:

1. **Empowerment and autonomy:** Self-help tactics enable women to take

an active role in their own mental health and well-being. By equipping women with practical tools and resources, they develop autonomy and agency in their lives, generating a better sense of control and empowerment.

2. **Accessibility and Affordability:** Professional treatment and medicine can be helpful resources, but they may not be available or inexpensive to everyone. Self-help initiatives provide a cost-effective and accessible option, allowing women to participate in therapeutic activities and practices at their speed and budget.

3. **Complementary to Professional Treatment:** Self-help tactics supplement professional treatment by offering extra support and reinforcement outside of therapy sessions. They can be valuable additions to established therapy modalities, increasing the efficacy of therapeutic procedures and facilitating long-term healing.

4. **Self-Awareness:** Participating in self-help activities promotes self-awareness and introspection, allowing women to better understand their ideas, emotions, and behaviors. Women who practice mindfulness and self-reflection might get insight into the root reasons for their depression and uncover appropriate coping techniques.

5. **Building Coping Skills:** Depression can present in a variety of ways, including feelings of hopelessness, low self-esteem, and difficulty coping with stress. Self-help tactics provide women with practical coping skills and resilience-building techniques to assist them in better negotiating these hurdles, allowing them to manage their symptoms and decrease the burden of depression in their everyday lives.

6. **Promotion of Holistic Well-being:** Self-help programs promote a holistic approach to well-being, addressing not only the psychological components of depression but also the physical, social, and spiritual dimensions of wellness. Women who incorporate lifestyle modifications such as exercise, nutrition, and social support can improve their general well-being and resilience in the face of depression.

7. **Long-Term Maintenance and Prevention:** Self-help strategies provide women with the tools and resources they need to maintain their mental

health over time and avoid relapses. Women can build resilience and protect themselves from future periods of depression by creating long-term self-care routines and engaging in continual self-monitoring.

4

2

Chapter One :Understanding Depression in Women

Definition and Overview of Depression

Depression is characterized by persistent feelings of melancholy, hopelessness, and a loss of interest or pleasure in formerly enjoyable activities. It is more than just feeling "down" or "blue"; it is an overwhelming sense of emptiness and despair that can last for weeks, months, or even years. Depression can take many different forms and severity levels, ranging from mild to severe, and can cause a variety of symptoms such as changes in appetite or weight, sleep disturbances, fatigue, feelings of worthlessness or guilt, and difficulty concentrating or making decisions.

An overview of symptoms

Depression symptoms vary greatly from person to person and may be impacted by age, gender, and personal circumstances. Common symptoms of depression are:

1. **Persistent emotions of melancholy or emptiness:** People suffering

from depression may feel a profound and pervasive sadness that endures despite efforts to alleviate it.

2. **Loss of interest or pleasure in activities:** Activities that were formerly enjoyable may no longer appeal to someone with depression, resulting in indifference or detachment from the world around them.

3. **Changes in appetite or weight:** Depression can affect appetite and eating habits, resulting in considerable weight changes, either through overeating or undereating.

4. **Sleep disturbances:** Insomnia or excessive sleeping are frequent signs of depression, which exacerbates feelings of exhaustion and lethargy.

5. **Fatigue or loss of energy:** Individuals with depression may experience persistent exhaustion, both physically and psychologically, making it difficult to engage in daily tasks.

6. **Feelings of worthlessness or excessive guilt:** Depression frequently results in bad self-perception, with people feeling unworthy of love, happiness, or achievement.

7. **Difficulty concentrating or making decisions:** Cognitive symptoms of depression can impair memory, attention, and executive functioning, making it difficult to concentrate or make choices.

8. **Thoughts of death or suicide:** In severe situations, depression can be accompanied by suicidal ideation as people try to find respite from their misery and despair.

Causes and Risk Factors

Depression has multiple causes, including genetic, biochemical, environmental, and psychological variables. While there is no one cause of depression, certain risk factors may raise the likelihood of getting the disorder, including:

- *A family history of depression or other mental health concerns.*
- *Traumatic life events, such as abuse, loss, or neglect.*
- *Chronic stress or adversity.*
- *Imbalanced brain chemistry or neurotransmitter function*

- ***Chronic illnesses and hormonal abnormalities are examples of medical problems.***
- ***Substance abuse or addiction.***

Diagnosis and Assessment

When diagnosing depression, it's important to consider symptoms, medical history, and psychosocial factors. Mental health professionals, such as psychiatrists, psychologists, and licensed therapists, may use standardized diagnostic criteria, such as those outlined in the Diagnostic and Statistical Manual of Mental Disorders (DSM-5), to determine whether an individual has a depressive disorder.

Treatment Approaches

Depression is often treated with a mix of psychotherapy, medication, and lifestyle adjustments. Psychotherapy, such as cognitive-behavioral therapy (CBT), interpersonal therapy (IPT), or psychodynamic therapy, can help people identify and challenge harmful thought patterns, learn coping skills, and enhance their interpersonal connections. Antidepressants and other medications may be taken to assist in balancing neurotransmitter levels in the brain and decrease depressive symptoms.

In addition to professional treatment, self-help activities such as exercise, relaxation techniques, mindfulness practices, and social support can be effective in controlling depression and improving general well-being. Lifestyle changes, such as eating a nutritious diet, exercising regularly, getting enough sleep, and avoiding alcohol and substance abuse, can all help to enhance mood and mental health.

Gender Differences in Depression

While depression can affect people of any gender, research has found several significant gender differences in the prevalence, presentation, and treatment of depression:

1. **Prevalence:** Studies consistently show that women are more likely than men to suffer from depression, with estimates indicating that women are roughly twice as likely as men to be diagnosed with depression during their lifetime. The gender disparity in depression prevalence begins in adolescence and persists into adulthood, with women experiencing higher rates of depression across all age groups.

2. **Presentation:** Men and women may experience similar symptoms of depression, such as persistent sadness, loss of interest or pleasure, and changes in appetite or sleep, but research suggests that women are more likely to experience certain symptoms, such as excessive guilt, rumination, and interpersonal sensitivity. Women may also be more likely to internalize their symptoms, which can lead to feelings of worthlessness or self-blame, whereas men may be more likely to externalize their symptoms through aggressive or substance-related behaviors.

3. **Risk Factors:** Biological, psychological, and social factors may all contribute to women's higher depression rates. Biological variables, such as hormonal variations associated with the menstrual cycle, pregnancy, childbirth, and menopause, may make women more susceptible to depression. Psychosocial factors, such as societal expectations, gender roles, and discrimination or trauma experiences, can all have an impact on women's mental health and contribute to depression.

4. **Treatment:** Gender variations in depression affect both treatment-seeking behavior and treatment outcomes. According to research, women may be more likely than men to seek help for depression and participate in mental health treatments such as therapy and medication. However, women may encounter additional challenges to seeking and receiving

quality mental health care, such as financial constraints, stigma, and a lack of social support. Furthermore, some studies suggest that women are more likely than men to experience side effects from antidepressants, necessitating different dosages or treatment strategies.

Cultural and Societal Influences

Cultural and societal influences, alongside biological and psychological factors, significantly impact gender differences in depression. Societal expectations of gender roles, relationships, and caregiving responsibilities can have an impact on women's mental health and contribute to depression. Women may face unique stressors and challenges, such as juggling multiple roles and responsibilities, achieving work-life balance, and encountering discrimination or marginalization based on gender, race, or socioeconomic status.

Furthermore, cultural norms and attitudes towards mental health may influence women's willingness to seek depression treatment, as well as their ability to access appropriate care. The stigma surrounding mental illness, as well as cultural beliefs about femininity, strength, and vulnerability, can create barriers to treatment and prevent women from receiving the support they need.

Empowering Women:

Addressing gender differences in depression requires a multifaceted approach that addresses the complex interplay of biological, psychological, social, and cultural factors. It is critical to raise awareness about the unique challenges that women face, as well as to promote gender-sensitive approaches to mental health care that consider women's varied experiences and needs. Empowering women to prioritize their mental health and seek help when needed is critical in reducing the burden of depression and promoting overall well-being. This may involve destigmatizing mental illness, providing education and resources about depression, and offering support and validation to women who are struggling.

Furthermore, addressing systemic inequities and promoting gender equality in all areas of life, including healthcare, education, and employment, can help create environments that support women's mental health and well-being. By challenging traditional gender norms, advocating for social justice, and promoting inclusive policies and practices, we can create a more equitable society where all individuals have the opportunity to thrive.

Common Symptoms and Signs in Women

Depression is a complex and multifaceted mental health illness defined by persistent feelings of sadness, hopelessness, and a loss of interest or pleasure in previously valued activities. While depression symptoms differ from person to person, there are a few typical markers that women may experience:

1. **Persistent Sadness or Emptiness:** One of the most distinguishing features of depression is a pervasive sense of sadness or emptiness that endures despite efforts to alleviate it. Women experiencing depression may experience feeling "stuck" in a black cloud or locked in a deep abyss of sadness.

2. **Loss of Interest or Pleasure:** Women who are depressed may lose interest in activities that were formerly fun or gratifying. Hobbies, social meetings, and even spending time with loved ones may seem like heavy tasks rather than sources of pleasure.

3. **Changes in Appetite or Weight:** Depression can affect appetite and eating patterns, resulting in severe weight changes. Some women may lose weight unintentionally due to a decrease in appetite, but others may gain weight by turning to food for comfort.

4. **Sleep Disorders:** Insomnia or excessive sleeping are common indicators of depression in women. Difficulty falling asleep, waking up repeatedly during the night, or waking up feeling unrefreshed can all worsen feelings of exhaustion and lethargy.

5. **Fatigue or Loss of Energy:** Women who are depressed may feel contin-

ually fatigued, both physically and psychologically. Even simple tasks might feel overwhelming, and getting out of bed in the morning may require a significant amount of effort.

6. **Feelings of Worthlessness or Excessive Guilt:** Depression frequently results in low self-perception, with women feeling unworthy of love, happiness, or achievement. They may have self-critical thoughts and dwell on past mistakes or perceived failures, creating a vicious cycle of self-blame and guilt.

7. **Difficulty Concentrating or Making Decisions:** Cognitive symptoms of depression can affect memory, attention, and executive function. Women may struggle to concentrate on work, make decisions, or retain key information, contributing to feelings of frustration and inadequacy.

8. **Physical Symptoms:** In addition to emotional and cognitive symptoms, depression can cause physical symptoms like headaches, digestive issues, and chronic pain. Women may develop unexplained aches and pains that may not respond to medication, complicating diagnosis and management.

Signs to Watch for

In addition to these frequent symptoms, there are several signals that a woman may be suffering from depression:

- **Withdrawal from Social Activities:** Women experiencing depression may withdraw from social activities, separating themselves from friends, family, and loved ones. They may cancel plans at the last minute, deny invitations to social gatherings, or avoid interaction with others completely.

- **Irritability or Mood fluctuations:** Although depression is commonly associated with feelings of melancholy or emptiness, some women may also experience irritability, agitation, or mood fluctuations. They may snap at loved ones, become quickly annoyed or angry, or struggle to maintain emotional control.

- **Changes in Appearance or Hygiene:** Depression can influence self-care behaviors, causing changes in appearance or hygiene. Women may overlook personal grooming routines such as washing, combing their hair, or changing their clothes regularly because they lack the motivation or energy to care for themselves.
- **Loss of Interest in Previously Enjoyed Activities:** Women who are depressed may lose interest in activities they used to enjoy or were enthusiastic about. Hobbies, interests, and pursuits that once brought delight may now feel meaningless or overpowering, causing a sensation of emptiness and alienation from their surroundings.
- **Difficulty Functioning in Daily Life:** Depression can impede a woman's capacity to function normally in everyday life. Simple activities like getting out of bed, going to work or school, or taking care of home responsibilities can seem impossible, leading to emotions of powerlessness and despair.
- **Thoughts of Death or Suicide:** In severe cases, depression may be accompanied by suicidal ideation. Women suffering from depression may express sentiments of hopelessness, worthlessness, or a desire to alleviate their agony through self-harm or death. It is critical to take any reference to suicide seriously and seek assistance promptly.

Myths and Misconceptions About Depression

Myth 1: Depression is simply a feeling of sadness.

One of the most common misconceptions regarding depression is that it is merely a passing melancholy. Depression is far more than simply feeling "blue" or "down." It is a complicated and devastating mental health illness marked by persistent emotions of melancholy, hopelessness, and despair that can last for weeks, months, or even years.

Depression has an impact on all aspects of a person's life, including their emotions, thoughts, physical health, and relationships. It is not something that can simply be "snapped out of" or overcome with determination. To manage effectively, however, compassionate understanding, support, and professional assistance are required.

Myth 2: Depression is an indication of weakness or personal failure.

Another widespread misconception regarding depression is that it is indicative of weakness or personal failure. This misperception contributes to the stigma around mental illness and stops many people from seeking assistance when they need it most.

Depression is not a character flaw or a sign of weakness; it is a medical disorder caused by a complex interaction of genetic, biochemical, environmental, and psychological variables. Depression can affect everyone, regardless of their strength, perseverance, or personal success.

Myth 3: People experiencing depression Just need to "Cheer Up" or "Get Over It"

Another detrimental myth regarding depression is that those suffering from it just need to "cheer up" or "get over it." This oversimplification ignores the enormous impact that depression may have on a person's life and downplays the significance of getting professional care and support.

Depression cannot be healed by optimistic thinking or simple lifestyle modifications. While self-care activities such as exercise, relaxation methods, and socializing can be beneficial, they should not replace evidence-based treatments like therapy and medication.

Myth 4: Depression only affects women.

While women are more likely than males to be diagnosed with depression, this does not imply that men are immune to the illness. Depression can afflict anyone of any gender, age, ethnicity, or origin; nevertheless, males may feel symptoms differently or be less likely to seek help owing to societal ideals of masculinity.

According to research, men may be more likely than women to have depression symptoms such as hostility, impatience, and substance addiction, rather than usual signals of sadness or tears. This variation in the presentation might make it difficult for males to recognize and acknowledge their symptoms, resulting in underdiagnosis and undertreatment.

Myth 5: Depression is only a phase that will pass on its own.

Another widespread misconception regarding depression is that it is merely a temporary state that will pass with time. While it is true that some people experience brief moments of melancholy or low mood, depression is a chronic and recurring mental health disease that requires professional attention and assistance to be effectively managed.

Ignoring or rejecting depression symptoms can worsen the disorder and have major repercussions, such as diminished functioning, relationship issues, and even suicide. If you or someone you love is suffering from depression, you must take the symptoms seriously and get help from a skilled mental health expert.

Myth 6: Antidepressants are the only treatments for depression.

Antidepressant medicines can be effective treatments for depression, but they are not the only alternative. Depression is a complicated and diverse disorder that may require a combination of therapy techniques to be effectively managed.

In addition to medication, psychotherapy, such as cognitive-behavioral therapy (CBT) or interpersonal therapy (IPT), can be extremely effective in addressing the root reasons of depression and establishing coping strategies to manage symptoms. Lifestyle changes, such as exercise, nutrition, and stress management skills, can all help to improve general mental health.

Myth 7: People with depression are always suicidal.

While suicidal ideation is a sign of sadness, not everyone who suffers from depression has thoughts of self-harm or suicide. Depression is a highly individualized disorder, with symptoms that vary greatly from person to person.

Some people with depression may have mild to moderate symptoms that can be managed with treatment and support, but others may have severe symptoms that greatly affect their functioning and quality of life. It is critical to recognize that depression exists on a continuum and to offer them support and understanding regardless of the intensity of their symptoms.

3

Chapter Two: The Impact of Depression on Women's Lives

Effects on Mental Health and Well-being

Mental health relates to our emotional, psychological, and social well-being, which includes our thoughts, feelings, and actions. It shapes how we think, feel, and act in response to life's problems, as well as our ability to deal with stress, form relationships, and make decisions. In contrast, mental well-being reflects our total sense of happiness, fulfillment, and life satisfaction.

When our mental health and well-being are strong, we are better able to deal with life's ups and downs, overcome hardship, and succeed in our personal and professional endeavors. However, when our mental health fails, the ramifications can be far-reaching, affecting all aspects of our lives.

Consequences of Poor Mental Health and Wellbeing

1. **Emotional distress:** Poor mental health can cause a wide range of emotional symptoms, including persistent sorrow, anxiety, irritation, aggression, and mood fluctuations. These feelings can be overwhelming

and uncontrollable, making it difficult to operate normally and sustain good relationships.

2. **Cognitive Impairment:** Mental health issues can impair cognitive function, reducing our capacity to think effectively, concentrate, make decisions, and solve problems. This can have an impact on our job or school performance, as well as our capacity to manage domestic activities and responsibilities.

3. **Physical Health Problems:** The mind-body connection is powerful, and poor mental health can have serious consequences for physical health. Chronic stress, anxiety, and depression have been related to a variety of physical health issues, including heart disease, gastrointestinal disorders, immune system failure, and chronic pain.

4. **Relationship Strain:** Mental health disorders can impact relationships with family members, friends, romantic partners, and colleagues, causing communication breakdowns, disputes, and trust to be impaired, leading to feelings of isolation, loneliness, and alienation.

5. **Work and Academic Performance:** Poor mental health can impact performance at work or school, resulting in lower productivity, absenteeism, and difficulties meeting deadlines or fulfilling duties. This can have an impact on career growth, academic performance, and overall job satisfaction.

6. **Substance Abuse:** Many people use alcohol, drugs, or other substances to relieve the symptoms of poor mental health. However, substance abuse can aggravate mental health issues, creating a vicious cycle of dependency and addiction.

7. **Social Withdrawal:** When dealing with poor mental health, people may withdraw from social activities and isolate themselves from others. This can intensify feelings of loneliness, melancholy, and anxiety, resulting in a vicious cycle of deteriorating mental health.

8. **Risk of Self-Harm or Suicide:** In extreme circumstances, poor mental health might raise the risk of self-harm or suicide. Feelings of hopelessness, worthlessness, and despair can become overwhelming, and people may consider suicide as the only option to relieve their suffering.

Promoting Mental Health and Well-being

Poor mental health can have a significant impact on our lives, but it's important to acknowledge that it's not fixed or unchanging. There are numerous steps we may take to enhance mental health and well-being while also building resilience in the face of hardship.

- **Self-Care:** Prioritise activities that nourish your mind, body, and spirit, such as exercise, nutrition, sleep, relaxation techniques, and enjoyable hobbies or interests.
- **Social Support:** Form supportive relationships with friends, family, and community people who can provide empathy, understanding, and encouragement during difficult times.
- **expert treatment:** If you are experiencing poor mental health, do not hesitate to seek treatment from a skilled mental health expert. Therapy, counseling, and medication can be quite helpful in treating mental health issues and improving overall well-being.
- **Stress Management:** Learn healthy coping techniques for stress, such as mindfulness meditation, deep breathing exercises, journaling, or participating in creative hobbies.
- **Boundaries:** Set healthy limits in your personal and professional lives to safeguard your mental and emotional well-being. Learn to say no to unreasonable demands or commitments, and instead prioritize things that bring you fulfillment and delight.
- **Meaning and Purpose:** Create a feeling of meaning and purpose in your life by making goals, following your hobbies, and participating in activities that reflect your values and beliefs.
- **thankfulness Practice:** Begin a daily practice of thankfulness by thinking about what you are grateful for in your life. Gratitude has been associated with enhanced mental health, resilience, and overall well-being.

Impact on Relationships and Social Life

- **Communication Breakdown:** Mental health difficulties can alter communication patterns, making it challenging to convey thoughts, feelings, and needs effectively. Individuals may struggle to express their emotions or withdraw completely from talks, resulting in misunderstandings, disputes, and feelings of irritation or resentment.
- **Emotional Distance:** Mental health issues can cause emotional distance between lovers, friends, and family members because people may feel disconnected or unable to connect with others on a deep emotional level. This emotional distance can strain relationships, eroding trust, intimacy, and closeness with time.
- **Increased Conflict:** Mental health issues can exacerbate conflict in relationships by causing heightened emotions, impatience, or mood swings, which contribute to disagreements, arguments, and tensions. Unresolved disputes can grow into feelings of anger, hatred, and isolation.
- **Carer Stress:** When one spouse or family member struggles with mental health concerns, the other may take on the position of carer, offering support, encouragement, and aid. While caregiving can be incredibly gratifying, it can also be emotionally stressful and physically exhausting, resulting in carer stress and burnout over time.
- **Codependency:** In some situations, mental health problems can lead to codependent tendencies in relationships, in which one partner becomes unduly reliant on the other for emotional support, validation, or stability. This dynamic can cause an imbalance of power and autonomy in the relationship, resulting in emotions of resentment, suffocation, or enablement.

Understanding the Impact of Social Life

- **Social retreat:** Mental health issues can contribute to social retreat because people may feel overwhelmed, apprehensive, or self-conscious in social circumstances. They may shun social meetings, parties, or activities entirely, preferring to isolate themselves from others rather than face imagined judgment or scrutiny from peers.

- **Loss of Interest:** Mental health issues can reduce excitement for previously appreciated social activities, hobbies, and pursuits. Individuals may lose motivation to engage in social relationships or struggle to get pleasure or satisfaction from socializing, resulting in feelings of indifference or alienation from the world around them.

- **Social Anxiety:** Mental health difficulties such as anxiety disorders can worsen social anxiety, making it difficult to interact with others or participate in social activities. Individuals may have significant dread or concern about socializing, resulting in avoidance behaviors or panic episodes in social situations.

- **Stigma and Discrimination:** Unfortunately, stigma and discrimination associated with mental illness can impede social inclusion and acceptance for those who are struggling. Individuals may be judged, prejudiced, or marginalized by peers, colleagues, or community members, causing feelings of humiliation, embarrassment, or isolation.

- **Impact on Friendships:** Friendships and social connections might suffer as a result of mental health issues, as people may struggle to maintain relationships or retreat from social contact entirely. Friends may feel unsure or uncomfortable about how to aid their hurting buddy, which can lead to feelings of powerlessness or inadequacy.

Strategies for Managing Relationships and Social Life

1. **Open Communication:** Encourage open and honest communication in your relationships, allowing each individual to express their thoughts, feelings, and needs without being judged or criticized. Engage in active listening and empathy, attempting to comprehend each other's perspectives and experiences.

2. **Mutual Support:** Provide support and encouragement to loved ones who are dealing with mental health challenges, remembering that support is a two-way street. Encourage open communication, acknowledge their

experiences, and provide practical support if needed, all while prioritizing your self-care and well-being.

3. **Boundaries:** Set appropriate boundaries in your relationships to protect your mental and emotional well-being. Communicate your wants and limits clearly and assertively, while respecting the boundaries of others. Setting limits can assist in reducing resentment, conflict, and burnout in relationships.

4. **Seek Professional Help:** If you or a loved one is experiencing mental health concerns, do not be afraid to seek treatment from a skilled mental health expert. Therapy, counseling, and medication can be quite helpful in treating mental health issues and improving overall well-being. A therapist can offer advice, support, and practical skills for managing relationships and social interactions.

5. **Practice self-care:** Prioritise self-care activities that nourish your mind, body, and spirit, such as exercise, proper nutrition, adequate sleep, relaxation techniques, and enjoyable hobbies or interests. Taking care of oneself allows you to be completely present in your relationships and social interactions, which promotes resilience and well-being.

6. **Build Support Networks:** Create a supportive network of friends, family, and peers who can provide empathy, understanding, and encouragement at difficult times. Join mental health support groups or online communities to connect with others facing similar issues.

Challenges in Work or Education

- **lower Productivity:** Mental health issues can impact concentration, focus, and motivation, resulting in lower productivity. Individuals may struggle to accomplish activities on time, fulfill deadlines, or maintain previous levels of performance. This can have an impact on job performance reviews, career promotion prospects, and overall job happiness.

- **Absenteeism:** Mental health disorders can lead to increased absenteeism at work because people may require time off to deal with symptoms such as anxiety, depression, or chronic stress. Frequent absences can interrupt production, damage relationships with coworkers, and provide issues for employers in terms of staffing and responsibility distribution.

- **Impaired Decision-Making:** Mental health issues can impair cognitive functioning, reducing a person's capacity to make decisions, solve problems, and think critically. This can have an impact on workplace decision-making processes, resulting in errors, misjudgments, and bad judgment calls that may have serious ramifications for both the individual and their coworkers.

- **Interpersonal Conflict:** Mental health difficulties can exacerbate interpersonal conflict in the workplace by causing individuals to experience heightened emotions, impatience, or mood swings, which can lead to conflicts, misunderstandings, and tension with coworkers and superiors. Conflict in the workplace can lead to a hostile work atmosphere, lower morale, and influence overall team cohesion and effectiveness.

- **Career Uncertainty:** Mental health issues can cause uncertainty and instability in a person's career path, since they may struggle to find consistent work or grow in their chosen sector. Fear of job loss, financial insecurity, or career losses can amplify emotions of worry, stress, and insecurity, negatively influencing mental health and well-being.

Understanding the Challenges of Education

- **Academic Performance:** Mental health issues can have an impact on academic achievement by impairing concentration, memory, and cognitive functioning. Students may fail to focus in class, complete work on time, or perform well on exams, resulting in lower marks, academic probation, or even dismissal in severe situations.

- **Attendance and engagement:** Mental health concerns can lead to higher absenteeism and lower engagement in educational activities because students may require time off to deal with symptoms such as anxiety, depression, or chronic stress. Students who miss courses, assignments, or tests may struggle to stay up with their homework and meet academic requirements.

- **Stress and Anxiety:** Academic expectations can worsen symptoms of stress and anxiety in individuals who are coping with mental health concerns. Pressure to achieve academically, meet deadlines, and manage various tasks can lead to emotions of overwhelm, perfectionism, and self-doubt, affecting mental health and well-being.

- **Social Isolation:** Mental health issues can lead to social disengagement and isolation in students, since they may feel overwhelmed, worried, or self-conscious in social circumstances. They may shun social gatherings, extracurricular activities, and campus events entirely, preferring to isolate themselves rather than face imagined judgment or scrutiny from peers.

- **Access to Support Services:** While many educational institutions provide counseling, therapy, or academic accommodations to students with mental health concerns, these services may be restricted or stigmatized. Students may be hesitant to seek help because they are concerned about confidentiality, judgment, or the perceived impact on their academic records or future professional opportunities.

Strategies for Navigating Challenges at Work or Education

1. **Open Communication:** Encourage open and honest conversations with your managers, coworkers, instructors, or academic advisors about your mental health issues and how they may be affecting your job or academic performance. Seek modifications or adaptations that can help you meet your mental health needs while still allowing you to carry out your obligations efficiently.

2. **Self-Care:** Prioritise activities that nourish your mind, body, and spirit, such as exercise, nutrition, sleep, relaxation techniques, and enjoyable hobbies or interests. Taking care of oneself enables you to actively participate in your work or school, promoting resilience and well-being.

3. **Seek Help:** If you are experiencing mental health difficulties, do not be afraid to seek help from mental health specialists, support groups, or peer networks. Therapy, counseling, and peer support can provide affirmation, encouragement, and practical techniques for dealing with

workplace or educational obstacles.

4. **Set realistic goals:** Set reasonable and attainable goals for yourself in your career or school, taking into account your mental health needs and limits. Break down larger jobs or projects into smaller, more manageable segments, and celebrate your accomplishments along the way.

5. **Advocate for Change:** Propose improvements to workplace or educational policies and practices that promote mental health and well-being for all people. This may involve pushing for better access to mental health resources, decreasing the stigma associated with mental illness, and fostering an environment of empathy, understanding, and support.

Coping with Stigma and Shame

Stigma refers to society's unfavorable attitudes, beliefs, and preconceptions about those with mental illnesses. This stigma can take many forms, including discrimination, prejudice, and social isolation. Misconceptions, fear, and a lack of knowledge are common causes of stigma in the mental health community, leading to widespread misunderstanding and the perpetuation of negative stereotypes.

Shame, on the other hand, is a deeply personal emotion triggered by feelings of inadequacy, unworthiness, or dishonor. Individuals may feel ashamed as a result of internalizing societal stigma or as a reaction to their own perceived flaws or challenges. The shame surrounding mental health may be especially insidious, undermining self-esteem, eroding self-worth, and preventing people from seeking the care and support they require.

Impact of Stigma and Shame

Stigma and shame around mental health can have a dramatic impact on every part of an individual's life.

- **Barriers to Seeking:** Stigma and shame can be substantial impediments to help-seeking behavior, stopping people from seeking support, therapy, or resources. Fear of being judged, rejected, or discriminated against may cause people to suffer in silence rather than seek the care they require to recover and heal.

- **Delayed Diagnosis and Treatment:** Stigma and shame associated with mental health can cause delayed diagnosis and treatment because people are hesitant to report their symptoms or seek professional care. This delay can prolong suffering, aggravate symptoms, and raise the chance of poor outcomes like hospitalization, self-harm, or suicide.
- **Social Isolation:** Stigma and shame can lead to social isolation and withdrawal when people are afraid of exposing their mental health issues to friends, family members, or peers. This isolation can aggravate emotions of loneliness, alienation, and despair, worsening mental health symptoms and lowering quality of life.
- **Impact on Relationships:** The stigma and guilt associated with mental health can damage relationships with friends, family members, and romantic partners. Individuals may be afraid of being judged or rejected by their loved ones, so they hide their problems or isolate themselves from those who care about them. This can result in a cycle of secrecy, mistrust, and emotional distance within partnerships.
- **Internalized Stigma:** People who have experienced stigma and shame related to mental health may internalize these negative attitudes, leading to feelings of self-blame, self-criticism, and uncertainty. Internalized stigma can lower self-esteem, diminish confidence, and reinforce feelings of worthlessness or inadequacy.

Strategies for Dealing with Stigma and Shame

1. **Education and awareness:** To combat stigma and misinformation regarding mental health, educate yourself and others about the realities of mental illness. Learn about the causes, symptoms, and treatments of many mental health issues, and then share accurate information with friends, family, and coworkers to foster understanding and empathy.
2. **Seek Support:** When things get tough, reach out to trustworthy friends,

family members, or support groups for empathy, understanding, and encouragement. Connecting with people who have had similar experiences can provide validation, validation, and support, reducing feelings of loneliness and shame.

3. **Practice self-compassion:** Cultivate self-compassion by treating oneself with love, understanding, and acceptance, particularly when dealing with stigma or shame related to mental health. Engage in self-care activities that nourish your mind, body, and soul, and counteract self-critical thoughts with positive statements and beliefs.

4. **Challenge Negative Beliefs:** Reframe negative assumptions and prejudices about mental health to provide positive and inspiring viewpoints. Recognize that mental illness is not a sign of weakness or personal failure, but rather a common and treatable health issue affecting millions of individuals throughout the world.

5. **Speak out:** Share your mental health experiences with others openly and honestly, breaking the silence and combating the stigma surrounding mental illnesses. Speaking up can help decrease the stigma and secrecy surrounding mental health, build empathy and understanding, and foster a culture of acceptance and support.

6. **Set boundaries:** Set appropriate boundaries with people or settings that promote stigma or shame around mental health. Surround yourself with individuals who encourage and validate your experiences, and avoid those who reject or downplay your challenges.

7. **Advocate for Change:** Support policy reforms, legislation, and initiatives that increase mental health awareness, education, and access to resources and support services. By pushing for systemic change, you may help break down institutional barriers and create a more inclusive and supportive environment for people with mental illnesses.

4

Chapter Three: Building Awareness and Seeking Help

Overcoming Barriers to Seeking Help

Seeking help for mental health difficulties may be a frightening and difficult process, with numerous challenges and barriers preventing many people from seeking help. These hurdles, whether caused by stigma, shame, financial restraints, or a lack of information, can exacerbate mental health issues and prevent people from receiving the care they require. In this in-depth examination, we will look at the numerous hurdles to getting mental health treatment and suggest practical solutions for overcoming them.

Understanding the barriers to seeking help

- **Stigma and Shame:** Many people are still hesitant to seek help because of the stigma and shame associated with mental health issues. Society's unfavorable attitudes, ideas, and prejudices about mental illness can cause humiliation, self-blame, and fear of judgment or discrimination, prompting people to suffer in silence rather than seek help.
- **Lack of Awareness:** Many people may be unaware of the signs and

symptoms of mental health issues, or they may fail to recognize when they are experiencing them. Individuals who lack a clear grasp of what constitutes mental illness and where to get help may struggle to recognize the need for treatment or may wait until symptoms worsen.

- **Financial Constraints:** Financial constraints can be substantial hurdles to getting mental health care, especially for people who do not have enough insurance or financial resources. Many people may find the cost of therapy, medication, or other mental health services prohibitively expensive, prompting them to forego treatment or rely on self-help measures.

- **Limited Access to Care:** Even for those who recognize the importance of mental health support, access to care can be hampered by variables such as geographic location, availability of mental health practitioners, or long wait times for appointments. Individuals in rural or underdeveloped locations may have difficulty accessing timely and effective mental health care due to a lack of resources.

- **Cultural and Linguistic Barriers:** Cultural and linguistic obstacles might also keep people from seeking treatment for mental health disorders. The cultural stigma associated with mental illness, language challenges, or skepticism of Western medical techniques may deter people from obtaining help from traditional mental health providers.

- **Fear of Diagnosis or Labelling:** Some people are afraid of being officially diagnosed with a mental health disorder or being labeled as "mentally ill." Individuals may avoid getting treatment or admitting their troubles to others due to a fear of being viewed as weak, imperfect, or abnormal, resulting in more isolation and pain.

- **Lack of Social Support:** Although social support is important in mental health rehabilitation, many people may not have supportive relationships or networks to turn to during stressful times. Feelings of loneliness, isolation, or detachment can exacerbate mental health issues and make it difficult for people to seek treatment.

Overcoming Barriers to Getting Help

1. **Education and awareness:** Increase your knowledge and comprehension of mental health concerns by educating yourself and others on the signs, symptoms, and treatment choices for common mental health conditions. Challenge stigma and preconceptions by sharing accurate information and personal stories that humanize mental illness while reducing shame and judgment.

2. **Normalise help-seeking behavior:** Normalise help-seeking behavior by encouraging open and honest discussions about mental health in your community, workplace, or social circles. Encourage others to share their stories and seek help when necessary, promoting an environment of acceptance, understanding, and support.

3. **Seek Affordable or Free options:** Look for mental health options in your town, such as community health centers, charitable organizations, or online support groups. Many organizations provide sliding-scale pricing or pro bono services to those with limited financial resources.

4. **Use Telehealth Services:** Take advantage of telehealth services, which offer easy and accessible ways to receive mental health care from the comfort of your own home. Many therapists and counselors provide virtual sessions through video conferencing technologies, making care more accessible regardless of physical location.

5. **Explore Self-Help Resources:** Look into self-help resources like books, websites, and mobile applications that provide evidence-based solutions for managing mental health problems. Self-help tools can provide essential knowledge, support, and coping skills to people who are unable or unable to seek conventional mental health care.

6. **Create a Support Network:** Create a support system of friends, family members, or peers who can provide empathy, understanding, and encouragement during difficult times. Connect with people who have had similar experiences by joining support groups or online communities where you may share information, stories, and coping tactics.

7. **Practice Self-Care:** Prioritise self-care activities that nourish your mind,

body, and spirit, such as exercise, nutrition, sleep, relaxation techniques, and enjoyable hobbies or interests. Taking care of yourself helps you cope with stress, manage symptoms, and preserve your general well-being.

8. **Challenge Negative Ideas:** Identify and challenge any negative or self-limiting ideas that are keeping you from obtaining help for mental health difficulties. Recognize that getting help demonstrates strength and courage, not weakness or failure and that you are entitled to support and compassion at difficult times.

Understanding the Importance of Self-Care

Self-care refers to a wide range of activities and practices that improve health, well-being, and resilience. It entails consciously prioritizing our own needs and promoting our physical, emotional, and mental well-being. Self-care is neither selfish nor indulgent; it is a necessary component of achieving balance and vigor in our lives.

Self-care can come in various forms, including:

1. **Physical Self-care:** Physical self-care entails taking care of our bodies through activities like exercise, the right nutrition, enough sleep, and frequent medical check-ups. It also entails maintaining proper hygiene, avoiding dangerous substances, and participating in activities that promote relaxation and renewal.

2. **Emotional Self-Care:** Emotional self-care entails looking after our emotional well-being and developing good relationships with ourselves and others. This may include expressing emotions in healthy ways, establishing boundaries, practicing self-compassion, and seeking help from friends, family members, or mental health experts as needed.

3. **Mental Self-Care:** Mental self-care entails promoting our cognitive and intellectual well-being through activities that stimulate and challenge the mind. Reading, learning new skills, indulging in creative hobbies, and practicing mindfulness and meditation can all help to improve brain clarity and attention.

4. **Spiritual Self-Care:** Spiritual self-care entails strengthening our connection to something larger than ourselves and discovering meaning and purpose in life. This could involve practicing meditation, prayer, or yoga, spending time in nature, or participating in activities that encourage introspection, gratitude, and spiritual growth.

The Importance of Self-Care

- **Stress Reduction:** Self-care routines such as exercise, relaxation techniques, and mindfulness meditation can assist in alleviating the physiological and psychological consequences of stress on the body and mind. By adding self-care into our daily routines, we may better cope with life's obstacles and stresses while also encouraging resilience in the face of hardship.
- **Improved Physical Health:** Prioritising physical self-care, such as regular exercise, the right nutrition, and adequate sleep, can have a variety of health benefits. Regular physical activity lowers the risk of chronic diseases like heart disease, diabetes, and obesity, while good nutrition and sleep promote immune function and overall health.
- **Enhanced Emotional Well-Being:** Emotional self-care activities like expressing emotions, setting boundaries, and seeking support from others can help us control our emotions and create a stronger sense of emotional well-being. Recognizing and honoring our emotions allows us to develop resilience and healthy connections with ourselves and others.
- **Enhanced Mental Clarity and Focus:** Mental self-care activities like reading, learning new skills, and practicing mindfulness meditation can help to sharpen cognitive functioning and increase mental clarity and focus. Giving our thoughts time to relax and recharge improves productivity, creativity, and problem-solving abilities.
- **Increased Self-Compassion and Self-Esteem:** Practicing self-compassion and self-care leads to a higher sense of self-worth and esteem. By putting our own needs first and treating ourselves with care and compassion, we may combat negative self-talk and build a more positive and caring inner

conversation.

- **Better Relationships:** When we prioritize self-care, we have more energy, patience, and empathy to put into our relationships with others. By prioritizing our own needs, we may be more present and real in our interactions with friends, family, and coworkers, resulting in stronger connections and more meaningful relationships.
- **Increased Resilience:** Self-care habits help us adapt and cope with life's obstacles. By investing in our physical, emotional, and mental well-being, we may recover faster from failures and hardship, navigating life's ups and downs with greater ease and grace.

Practical Strategies for Self-Care

1. **Prioritize your needs:** Take the time to analyze your requirements and prioritize activities and practices that will benefit your body, mind, and soul. Set boundaries for your time and energy, and don't be afraid to decline activities or obligations that exhaust you or hinder your well-being.
2. **Schedule self-care activities:** Include self-care activities in your daily or weekly agenda, just like any other important appointment or commitment. Make self-care a non-negotiable element of your routine, whether it's scheduling regular exercise, carving out time for relaxation, or participating in a pastime you enjoy.
3. **Practice Mindfulness:** Bring awareness to the present moment and tune into your thoughts, feelings, and sensations without judgment. Meditation, deep breathing, and body scan exercises are all examples of mindfulness activities that can aid with stress reduction, self-awareness, and emotional well-being.
4. **Nurture your relationships:** Invest in healthy and supporting connections with friends, family, and loved ones who inspire and motivate you. Make time for genuine interactions, whether through phone conversations, social outings, or shared hobbies that you enjoy.
5. **Set realistic goals:** Set realistic and attainable goals for yourself, taking

into account your present skills, resources, and priorities. Break down huge ambitions into smaller, more doable steps and celebrate your accomplishments along the way. Be kind to yourself and practice self-compassion, even if things don't go as planned.

6. **Engage in activities that bring you joy:** Make time for activities and hobbies that you enjoy, such as reading, listening to music, gardening, or spending time outside. Engaging in activities that nourish your spirit and give you pleasure is an important part of self-care.

7. **Seek Help When You Need It:** If you need help, don't be afraid to ask friends, family members, or mental health experts. If you're having trouble with your mental health, get help and support from someone you trust, or try therapy or counseling to examine your emotions and create coping methods.

Finding Support Systems and Resources

Support systems are a network of people, organizations, and resources that offer emotional, practical, and informational assistance to people suffering from mental health issues. These support systems may include:

- **Personal Support:** Personal support refers to friends, family members, romantic partners, and other personal ties that provide empathy, understanding, and encouragement during difficult times. Personal support networks create a sense of belonging and connection, making people feel valued and supported.
- **Professional Support:** Mental health specialists such as therapists, counselors, psychologists, and psychiatrists offer clinical expertise, assessment, and treatment for mental health problems. These experts provide evidence-based interventions including therapy, medication management, and psychiatric care to assist people in managing their symptoms and enhancing their overall well-being.
- **Peer Support:** Peer assistance entails connecting with individuals who share similar life experiences with mental health issues. Peer support

groups, internet forums, and community organizations allow people to share their stories, receive affirmation, and exchange practical advice and coping tactics with others who understand their problems.

- **Community Support:** Community support refers to local organizations, nonprofits, and grassroots initiatives that offer mental health education, advocacy, and services to individuals and families in need. These organizations may provide support groups, workshops, helplines, or referral services to help people find the resources and support they need.
- **Online Resources:** Websites, mobile apps, and digital platforms provide information, tools, and support for mental health challenges. Self-help materials, interactive tools, virtual treatment platforms, and peer support forums are all examples of online services that allow people to get help from anywhere.

Importance of Support Systems

1. **Validation & Understanding:** Support systems provide validation and understanding by recognizing and affirming people's experiences with mental health issues. Connecting with others who share similar experiences helps to minimize feelings of loneliness and stigma while also fostering a sense of belonging and acceptance.
2. **Emotional Support:** Support networks provide emotional support by creating a secure area in which people can share their thoughts, concerns, and challenges without being judged. Emotional support from friends, family, or peers makes people feel heard, understood, and valued, which reduces feelings of loneliness and despair.
3. **Practical Assistance:** Support systems help people manage the problems of daily life, such as accessing healthcare services, managing medicines, and meeting necessities. Practical aid from friends, family, or community organizations reduces stress while promoting stability and self-sufficiency.
4. **Information and Education:** Support systems offer information and education on mental health challenges, treatment alternatives, and rele-

vant resources. Individuals who have access to accurate and trustworthy information are better equipped to make educated decisions about their care and successfully advocate for themselves.

5. **Coping Strategies and Skills:** Support systems provide individuals with coping strategies and skills to effectively manage their mental health difficulties. Peer support groups, therapy sessions, and online resources offer practical advice, coping tactics, and self-care measures to help people build resilience and well-being.

Finding Support Systems and Resources

- **Identify your needs:** When seeking mental health care, take the time to establish your specific needs and preferences. Consider the type of support you are searching for (e.g., emotional support, practical aid, peer connection) as well as the specific issues you are experiencing.
- **Reach out to personal support networks:** Begin by contacting friends, family members, or trustworthy folks in your support network. Share your thoughts and feelings openly and honestly, and let them know how they can help you through difficult situations.
- **Consider Professional Support:** Seek professional help from mental health specialists such as therapists, counsellors, or psychiatrists. To find the best fit for you, research local providers, read reviews, and book first consultations.
- **Explore Peer Support Options:** Consider peer assistance options such as support groups, online forums, or community organizations that cater to people with similar mental health difficulties. Connect with other people who understand your situation and can provide empathy, affirmation, and practical guidance.
- **Access Community Resources:** Look into local community resources, NGOs, or grassroots organizations that provide mental health assistance and resources. Attend local support groups, workshops, or events to interact with others while also gaining access to vital information and resources.

- **Use Online Resources:** Use online resources including websites, mobile applications, and digital platforms to get knowledge, tools, and support for your mental health. Look through self-help materials, interactive tools, and virtual therapy choices to locate resources that match your requirements.
- **Advocate for yourself:** As a person dealing with mental health issues, you have the right to advocate for your needs. Don't be hesitant to speak out and ask for the assistance and adjustments you require to prosper. Advocate for changes in your community's policies, practices, and attitudes to increase mental health understanding and acceptance.

Chapter Four: Strategies for Managing Depression

Incorporating Mindfulness and Relaxation Techniques

Mindfulness is the discipline of paying full attention to the present moment with openness, curiosity, and acceptance. It entails paying attention to your thoughts, feelings, sensations, and surroundings without judgment, as well as developing a better sense of awareness and presence in your daily life.

Relaxation, on the other hand, entails purposefully releasing tension from the body and mind, resulting in a sense of serenity, ease, and tranquillity. Relaxation techniques aim to trigger the body's natural relaxation response, which reduces the physiological and psychological impacts of stress while also boosting physical and mental well-being.

Benefits of Mindfulness and Relaxation

1. **Stress Reduction:** Mindfulness and relaxation practices are effective tools for reducing stress and increasing relaxation. By bringing awareness to the present moment and releasing tension from the body and

mind, these activities trigger the body's relaxation response, which counteracts the physiological and psychological impacts of stress.

2. **Improved Emotional Well-Being:** Mindfulness and relaxation techniques can improve emotional well-being by increasing self-awareness, emotional control, and resilience. These practices help people handle unpleasant emotions more efficiently while also building a greater feeling of presence and acceptance.

3. **Enhanced Cognitive Functioning:** Mindfulness activities have been demonstrated to improve cognitive functions, such as attention, memory, and problem-solving skills. Mindfulness enhances cognitive clarity and mental agility by teaching the mind to focus on the present moment and avoid distractions, resulting in increased productivity and creativity.

4. **Better Sleep Quality:** Mindfulness and relaxation techniques can help you sleep better by boosting calm and lowering anxiety and tension. Deep breathing, progressive muscle relaxation, and guided imagery can all assist in relaxing the nervous system and prepare the body and mind for a good night's sleep.

5. **Increased Self-Compassion:** Mindfulness techniques create increased self-compassion by helping people to be compassionate, accept themselves, and avoid judgment. Individuals who have a more sympathetic approach towards themselves might lessen self-criticism while also increasing their sense of self-worth and self-esteem.

Incorporating Mindfulness and Relaxation Techniques into Your Daily Life

- **Begin with Small Steps:** Begin implementing mindfulness and relaxation practices into your routine by taking tiny, attainable steps. Set aside a few minutes per day to practice mindfulness or relaxation, gradually increasing the time as you get more comfortable with the techniques.

- **Practice Mindful Breathing:** Mindful Breathing is one of the most easy and accessible mindfulness activities. Spend a few moments each day focusing on your breath, experiencing the sensations of inhaling and exhaling without attempting to change or control them. This technique helps you focus on the present moment and promotes calm.

- **Engage in Daily Mindful Activities:** Incorporate mindfulness into your daily routine by paying attention to your senses and being completely engaged in the present moment. Pay attention to the sights, sounds, smells, tastes, and feelings around you when eating, walking, or doing dishes to develop a stronger sense of presence and appreciation for the present moment.

- **Practice Progressive Muscle Relaxation:** Progressive Muscle Relaxation is a relaxation technique that involves gradually tensing and relaxing muscle groups throughout the body. Start by tensing a specific muscle area (e.g., your shoulders) for a few seconds, then release the tension and notice how relaxed you feel. Repeat this method with each muscle group, gradually making your way around the body.

- **Incorporate Mindful Movement:** Try mindful movement techniques like yoga, tai chi, or qigong, which combine light physical activity with mindfulness and breath awareness. These techniques encourage relaxation, flexibility, and balance while also increasing mind–body awareness and connection.

- **Practice guided imagery:** Guided imagery is a relaxing technique in which you imagine a serene and calming environment or scenario in great detail. Close your eyes and envision yourself in a peaceful and relaxing setting, such as a beach, forest, or alpine meadow. Relax and unwind by focusing on the sights, sounds, smells, and sensations of this fictional area.

- **Create a relaxation ritual:** Create a relaxing ritual or routine that you can work into your daily or weekly schedule. Whether it's taking a warm bath, listening to calming music, or practicing meditation before bed, discover things that help you decompress and encourage relaxation and incorporate them into your normal routine.

- **Be patient and persistent:** Remember that implementing mindfulness and relaxation practices into your everyday routine is a gradual process that requires patience and effort. Be patient with yourself and tenacious in your efforts, and don't be disheartened by setbacks or obstacles along the way. With time and persistence, you'll start to see the benefits of these habits in your everyday life.

Nurturing Positive Relationships

Humans are fundamentally sociable creatures that want connection and belonging. Positive relationships are crucial to our well-being, influencing our happiness, health, and general quality of life. Nurturing strong relationships, whether with friends, family, love partners, or coworkers, enhances our lives and gives us critical support, understanding, and companionship.

The significance of positive relationships

Positive connections are vital for our well-being, as they influence numerous facets of our lives.

1. **Emotional Support:** Positive relationships offer emotional support during times of stress, struggle, or uncertainty. Knowing that we can turn to others for support, encouragement, and understanding strengthens our resilience and ability to deal with life's obstacles.
2. **Social Connection:** Positive interactions promote a sense of social connection and belonging, which alleviates feelings of loneliness, isolation, and alienation. Having a network of friends, family members, and loved ones with whom we can share our experiences, interests, and values helps us feel more connected to others.
3. **Physical Health:** Positive relationships have been related to enhanced physical health outcomes such as lower blood pressure, a lower chance of chronic diseases, and greater immunological function. Positive relationships provide emotional support and companionship, which helps to reduce stress and improve general health and well-being.
4. **Mental Health:** Positive connections promote mental health and emotional well-being. Feeling loved, supported, and understood by others boosts our self-esteem, lowers anxiety and sadness, and promotes a

stronger sense of happiness and life satisfaction.

5. **Personal Development:** Positive interactions allow us to grow as individuals, find ourselves, and enhance our lives. Interacting with people with various ideas, abilities, and experiences broadens our horizons, tests our preconceptions, and motivates us to learn and evolve as individuals.

Qualities of Positive Relationships

Positive relationships have several aspects that contribute to their strength and persistence.

1. **Trust and respect:** Trust and respect are the building blocks of effective relationships, fostering a secure and supportive environment in which people feel valued, accepted, and understood. Building trust and respect necessitates honesty, dependability, and mutual respect for one another's boundaries and autonomy.

2. **Communication and Openness:** Effective communication and openness are critical to maintaining positive relationships. Active listening, empathy, and the honest expression of thoughts, feelings, and needs are all essential components of healthy communication. Openness enables people to communicate openly and honestly with one another, creating understanding and connection.

3. **Empathy and Compassion:** Empathy and compassion are essential components of effective relationships, allowing people to understand and respond to one another's feelings with care and delicacy. Empathy is noticing and validating others' perspectives, whereas compassion entails providing assistance and kindness in times of need.

4. **Mutual Support and Encouragement:** Positive relationships include mutual support and encouragement, with persons offering emotional, practical, and instrumental assistance as needed. Supporting one other's goals, objectives, and well-being develops relationships and fosters a sense of teamwork and collaboration.

5. **Shared Values and Interests:** Positive relationships are frequently based

on common values, interests, and experiences that bring people together and build a sense of connection and belonging. Individuals' bonds are strengthened when they share common goals, hobbies, or values. This also allows for shared experiences and enjoyment.

Practical Strategies for Developing Positive Relationships

- **Prioritise quality time together:** Make time for meaningful conversations and activities with your loved ones, such as eating together, going for a stroll, or simply spending time at home. Prioritizing quality time allows you to develop your bonds and make memorable experiences together.
- **Practice Active Listening:** Active listening involves paying complete attention to the speaker, maintaining eye contact, and expressing genuine interest in what they have to say. Listen without interrupting or criticizing, and then reflect on what you've heard to ensure comprehension and validation.
- **Express Appreciation and Gratitude:** Thank the people in your life for their contributions, strengths, and traits. Take the time to show your thanks with words, gestures, or acts of kindness, letting them know how much you value and appreciate them.
- **Constructive Conflict Resolution:** Address conflicts and disagreements positively and respectfully, with an emphasis on finding solutions rather than assigning blame or escalating the situation. Use active listening, empathy, and compromise to create a solution that pleases both sides and enhances the relationship.
- **Show Affection and Support:** Express your love and support for your loved ones through physical touch, words of affirmation, and acts of kindness. Provide encouragement, affirmation, and comfort when needed, and enjoy their victories and accomplishments together.
- **Foster mutual growth and development:** Encourage reciprocal growth and development by supporting one another's goals, desires, and personal growth journeys. Provide constructive comments, encouragement, and accountability to assist each other in realizing your greatest potential and

realizing your aspirations.

- **Respect each other's boundaries:** Respect each other's boundaries, preferences, and autonomy while communicating freely and honestly about your needs and limitations. Create a friendly and courteous environment in which people feel free to express themselves and enforce their limits without fear of being judged or criticized.
- **Develop positive communication patterns:** Develop great communication habits by using assertiveness, empathy, and active listening in your interactions with others. Use "I" expressions to express your thoughts and feelings, rather than blaming or criticising others. Concentrate on establishing common ground and comprehending each other's viewpoints.

Setting Realistic Goals and Priorities

Goal setting is the process of selecting precise objectives or aims that we wish to achieve within a given time frame. Goals give direction, focus, and drive, directing our actions and decisions toward the intended results. Setting objectives, whether in a personal or professional environment, allows us to clarify our aims, track progress, and celebrate successes along the way.

However, not all aims are equal. Setting unrealistic or too-ambitious objectives can cause dissatisfaction, fatigue, and disappointment, eroding our confidence and enthusiasm. As a result, it is critical to establish goals that are hard yet attainable, consistent with our values and priorities, and foster growth and development.

The significance of establishing realistic goals and priorities

- **Clarity and focus:** Setting realistic goals and priorities provides clarity and focus, allowing us to identify what is most important and where we should put our time, energy, and resources. By identifying clear objectives and priorities, we may streamline our efforts and eliminate distractions or detours that could impede our success.
- **Motivation and Commitment:** Setting realistic goals and priorities fuels

motivation and commitment, pushing us to take action and persevere in the face of obstacles. When we believe our objectives are feasible and important, we are more likely to remain motivated and committed to accomplishing them, even when challenges come.

- **Sustainable Progress:** Realistic goals and priorities enhance long-term success and enable us to make steady and gradual progress toward our objectives. Setting reasonable goals and pacing ourselves appropriately allows us to retain momentum while avoiding burnout or tiredness along the way.
- **Flexibility and Adaptability:** Setting realistic goals and priorities promotes flexibility and adaptation, allowing us to alter our plans and methods as necessary in response to changing circumstances or unanticipated problems. Flexibility allows us to stay nimble and adaptable while pursuing our goals, rather than becoming rigid or fixed on a predetermined path.
- **Enhanced Well-Being:** Setting realistic goals and priorities improves our general well-being by encouraging balance, fulfillment, and pleasure in our lives. When our goals are aligned with our values and priorities, we feel more connected and purposeful, which leads to more happiness and fulfillment.

Practical Strategies for Creating Realistic Goals and Priorities

1. **Reflect on your values and priorities:** Start by reflecting on your values, passions, and long-term goals. Consider what is most important to you in life, both personally and professionally, and determine where you want to devote your time and attention. Use this reflection as a starting point for developing goals and priorities that are consistent with your values and contribute to your overall well-being and fulfillment.
2. **Set SMART Goals:** Use the SMART criteria to create goals that are specific, measurable, achievable, relevant, and time-constrained. Specific objectives are clear and well-defined; measurable goals are quantifiable and trackable; achievable goals are reasonable and reachable; relevant

goals are in line with your values and priorities; and time-bound goals have a set completion date.

3. **Break Down Goals into Manageable Steps:** Divide larger goals into smaller, more manageable steps or milestones that you may work on incrementally. Breaking down goals into smaller tasks makes them more achievable and less intimidating, helping you to make consistent progress and stay inspired along the way.

4. **Prioritise Goals Based on Importance and Urgency:** Prioritise your goals in order of importance and urgency, focusing on those that will have the most impact on your long-term success and well-being. Use the Eisenhower Matrix and other priority-setting frameworks to identify high-priority tasks and spend your time and resources accordingly.

5. **Be Realistic and Flexible:** Be realistic about your ability to complete tasks within a certain timeframe, and be open to changing your goals and priorities as needed. Recognize that conditions might change and unforeseen obstacles can develop, forcing you to adjust your plans and strategy accordingly. Accept flexibility and resilience in pursuit of your goals, and be willing to change your strategy when circumstances change.

6. **Monitor Progress and Adjust as Needed:** Keep track of your progress toward your goals and compare your performance to established milestones or benchmarks. Celebrate your accomplishments and milestones along the road, and use comments to find areas for improvement or change. Be proactive in making course changes as needed to keep on track and sustain momentum toward your goals.

7. **Practice Self-Compassion and Patience:** Throughout the goal-setting process, remember that failures and obstacles are a normal part of growth and development. If things don't go as planned, be gentle and helpful to yourself, and try not to criticize or talk negatively about yourself. Remember that growth takes time, and success is frequently the product of determination and endurance in the face of adversity.

8. **Seek Support and Accountability:** Seek out friends, family members, mentors, or colleagues who can offer encouragement, guidance, and accountability as you work towards your objectives. Share your goals with

others and request their help in keeping you accountable and motivated along the road.

Chapter Five: Lifestyle Changes for Better Mental Health

Importance of Nutrition and Exercise

Nutrition is the process by which the body absorbs and uses nutrients from meals to promote growth, repair, and important functions. A well-balanced diet has all of the important elements that the body requires to survive, including carbs, proteins, fats, vitamins, minerals, and water. Proper nutrition is important for:

- **Physical Health:** A nutritious diet promotes excellent physical health by supplying the body with the energy and nutrients it requires to perform properly. Nutrient-dense diets nourish muscles, bones, organs, and tissues, hence promoting growth, repair, and immunological function.
- **Disease Prevention:** A balanced diet can help prevent many chronic diseases, such as heart disease, diabetes, obesity, and some malignancies. Fruits, vegetables, whole grains, and lean proteins are nutrient-dense foods that contain antioxidants, fiber, and other chemicals that help to prevent oxidative stress and inflammation.

- **Energy and Vitality:** Proper nutrition provides the body with energy, vitality, and stamina, improving physical performance, endurance, and overall vitality. Nutrient-dense diets give a continuous flow of energy throughout the day, promoting mental focus, productivity, and alertness.
- **Mental Health:** Nutrition has a huge impact on mental health and emotional well-being. According to research, a nutritious diet rich in fruits, vegetables, whole grains, and omega-3 fatty acids may lower the risk of depression, anxiety, and other mood disorders while also improving cognitive performance and emotional resilience.
- **Weight Management:** A well-balanced diet promotes healthy weight management by supplying needed nutrients while moderating desire and cravings. Nutrient-dense foods are more filling and fulfilling, lowering the risk of overeating and encouraging weight loss or maintenance.

The Importance of Exercise

Exercise is essential for improving cardiovascular health, flexibility, and strength by engaging the body's muscles. Regular exercise has various advantages for physical, mental, and emotional health, including:

- **Physical Fitness:** Regular exercise boosts cardiovascular health, muscular strength, endurance, and flexibility. Aerobic activity, like walking, running, swimming, or cycling, strengthens the heart and lungs, whereas strength training increases muscle mass and bone density.
- **Weight Management:** Exercise is essential for weight management since it burns calories, increases metabolism, and promotes fat loss. Both aerobic exercise and strength training increase calorie expenditure and metabolic rate, which aids in weight loss or maintenance.
- **Disease Prevention:** Regular exercise lowers the risk of chronic diseases such as heart disease, stroke, type 2 diabetes, and cancer. Physical activity promotes blood circulation, decreases blood pressure and cholesterol, and boosts immune function, lowering the risk of acquiring chronic health issues.

- **Mental Health:** Exercise has a significant impact on mental health and emotional well-being, lowering stress, anxiety, and depression. Physical activity increases the release of endorphins, neurotransmitters that promote enjoyment and relaxation while also increasing sleep quality and cognitive performance.
- **Stress Reduction:** Exercise is an excellent stress reliever, helping to alleviate the physiological and psychological consequences of stress on both body and mind. Physical activity causes the production of stress-relieving hormones such as endorphins and serotonin, as well as giving a healthy outlet for pent-up tension and irritation.

Practical Strategies for Integrating Nutrition and Exercise into Your Daily Life

1. **Prioritise nutrient-dense foods:** Include more nutrient-dense foods in your diet, such as fruits, vegetables, whole grains, lean meats, and healthy fats. Choose a range of colors, flavors, and textures to guarantee a well-balanced intake of key nutrients.
2. **Plan and prepare meals:** Make the effort to plan and prepare nutritious meals and snacks ahead of time, rather than relying on convenience or fast food. Batch cooking, meal planning, and stockpiling healthy staples can help you maintain a healthful diet even when you're busy.
3. **Stay Hydrated:** Drink plenty of water throughout the day to stay hydrated and improve your overall health and wellness. Water is vital for digestion, circulation, temperature regulation, and nutrient transfer, so strive to drink at least 8-10 glasses per day.
4. **Listen to your body:** Pay attention to your body's hunger and fullness signals, and eat thoughtfully to fuel yourself naturally. Focus on eating when you're hungry, stopping when you're full, and selecting foods that make you feel energized and content.
5. **Include Physical Activity in Your Routine:** Find ways to include physical activity into your daily routine, whether through planned workouts, energetic hobbies, or ordinary activities. Aim for at least 150 minutes of

moderate-intensity aerobic activity or 75 minutes of vigorous-intensity aerobic activity per week, with muscle-strengthening activities on two or more days.

6. **Choose activities that you enjoy:** Choose physical activities that you enjoy and look forward to, such as walking, dancing, cycling, or playing sports. Finding activities that make you happy and satisfied helps you stay motivated and dedicated to regular exercise.

7. **Be consistent and persistent:** Make physical activity and nutritious nutrition a regular part of your daily routine, rather than sporadic or infrequent attempts. Consistency is essential for achieving results and preserving long-term health and well-being, so prioritize exercise and diet in your life.

8. **Set realistic goals and celebrate your achievements:** Set realistic and attainable objectives for both eating and activity and celebrate your accomplishments along the way. Whether you're accomplishing a fitness goal, attempting a new healthy recipe, or simply making healthier choices every day, take the time to recognize and celebrate your accomplishments.

Getting Adequate Sleep and Rest

Sleep is a naturally occurring condition of reduced consciousness and physical activity, marked by altered brain activity and decreased sensory awareness. During sleep, the body goes through important processes that facilitate physical restoration, cognitive consolidation, and emotional stability. In contrast, rest refers to moments of relaxation and recovery during which the body and mind can recharge and replenish.

Sleep and rest are both essential for overall health and well-being, supporting a variety of physiological and psychological processes.

- **Physical Recovery:** Sleep and rest allow the body to heal tissues, replenish energy stores, and regulate important physical systems. During sleep, the body produces growth hormones, repairs cellular damage, and boosts the immune system, which aids in physical recovery and regeneration.

- **Cognitive Functioning:** Sleep is crucial for cognitive functioning, memory consolidation, and information processing. Adequate sleep improves learning, problem-solving, and decision-making abilities while also encouraging creativity, attention, and mental clarity.
- **Emotional management:** Sleep and rest are critical for emotional management and psychological health. Adequate sleep regulates mood, reduces stress, and boosts emotional resilience, whereas insufficient sleep can cause irritation, anxiety, and mood swings.
- **Hormonal Balance:** Sleep and rest are essential for controlling hunger, metabolism, and stress response. Adequate sleep promotes the production of hormones like leptin and ghrelin, which control hunger and satiety, while also controlling cortisol levels and lowering the risk of stress-related illnesses.
- **immunological Function:** Sleep and rest are essential for good immunological function and disease resistance. During sleep, the body creates cytokines and antibodies to fight infection and inflammation while also encouraging tissue repair and healing.

The Importance of Getting Enough Sleep and Rest

1. **Physical Health:** Adequate sleep and rest are required to sustain physical health and vigor. Chronic sleep deprivation and insufficient rest have been related to a higher risk of obesity, diabetes, heart disease, and other chronic health problems. Getting enough sleep and rest improves general immune function, lowers inflammation, and promotes cardiovascular health.
2. **Mental Clarity:** Sleep and rest are necessary for mental clarity, focus, and cognitive performance. Sleep deprivation can affect memory, focus, and decision-making skills, resulting in lower productivity and performance. Adequate sleep and rest improve cognitive function, problem-solving abilities, and creativity.
3. **Emotional Well-Being:** Sleep and relaxation are essential for emotional

control and psychological health. Adequate sleep regulates mood, reduces stress, and boosts resilience to unpleasant emotions. Insufficient sleep, on the other hand, might cause irritation, anxiety, and mood changes.

4. **Stress Reduction:** Sleep and rest are effective stress relievers, lowering cortisol levels and promoting relaxation and renewal. Adequate sleep and rest enable the body to recuperate from the physiological and psychological impacts of stress, hence increasing resilience and coping abilities.

5. **Immune Function:** Sleep and rest are critical for keeping a healthy immune system and fighting infections and illnesses. During sleep, the body creates cytokines and antibodies that aid in the fight against pathogens and improve immunological function. Chronic sleep deprivation impairs immune function, making you more susceptible to infections and illnesses.

Practical Strategies for Getting Enough Sleep and Rest

1. **Make Sleep a Priority:** Establish a consistent sleep schedule and develop a calming nighttime routine. Aim for 7-9 hours of quality sleep per night, and try to go to bed and get up at the same time every day, including weekends.

2. **Create a Restful Environment:** Create a relaxing and sleep-friendly environment. Keep your bedroom cold, dark, and quiet, and invest in a comfortable mattress and pillows to promote good sleep. Reduce the amount of noise, light, and electronic devices that can interfere with your sleep, and consider utilizing white noise machines or earplugs to block out distractions.

3. **Practice relaxation techniques:** Incorporate relaxation techniques like deep breathing, meditation, or progressive muscle relaxation into your evening routine to help you relax and prepare for sleep. Relaxation practices can assist in relieving stress, calming the mind, and promoting restful sleep.

4. **Limit stimulants and electronics:** Limit your intake of coffee, nicotine, and alcohol, especially in the hours coming up to bedtime, as these can all interfere with sleep quality and length. Additionally, limit your screen time and exposure to electronic gadgets before bed, as the blue light released by displays can disrupt circadian cycles and interfere with sleep.

5. **Establish a Bedtime Routine:** Create a peaceful nighttime routine that tells your body it's time to unwind and prepare for sleep. Before going to bed, engage in relaxing activities like reading, having a warm bath, or listening to soothing music to induce relaxation and notify your body that it's time to sleep.

6. **Practice Good Sleep Hygiene:** Develop healthy routines and behaviors that support peaceful sleep. Avoid stimulating activities, big meals, and strenuous exercise before bedtime, and create a relaxing sleep environment.

7. **Stress Management:** Techniques like mindfulness, yoga, and journaling can help you manage your stress levels. Chronic stress can interfere with the quality and length of sleep, so learning good stress management techniques can help you sleep better and feel better overall.

8. **Seek Professional Help if Necessary:** If you continue to have problems sleeping despite applying these measures, consult a healthcare provider or sleep specialist. Chronic sleep issues may suggest an underlying sleep disorder or medical condition that necessitates treatment, so do not hesitate to seek professional advice and assistance.

Managing Stress and Avoiding Burnout

Stress is the body's natural response to demands or challenges, causing a series of physiological and psychological processes that aid in our ability to cope with dangers or pressure. While acute stress can be beneficial in some instances, chronic or long-term stress can be harmful to our health and well-being. Work-related stresses, interpersonal troubles, financial concerns, health issues, and big life transitions are all common causes of stress.

The Effects of Stress on Health and Well-Being

Chronic stress can have a dramatic impact on our physical, emotional, and mental health, causing a wide range of symptoms and health concerns, including:

- **Physical Health:** Chronic stress can weaken the immune system, raise the risk of cardiovascular disease, worsen pre-existing health conditions, and cause symptoms such as headaches, muscular tension, exhaustion, and gastrointestinal issues.
- **Emotional Well-Being:** Stress can hurt our emotional health, causing anxiety, irritation, mood swings, and sadness. Chronic stress can also hinder our capacity to deal with difficult situations, control emotions, and maintain strong relationships.
- **Mental Health:** Prolonged stress increases the likelihood of developing mental health illnesses such as anxiety disorders, depression, and post-traumatic stress disorder (PTSD). Chronic stress can exacerbate pre-existing mental health disorders and worsen symptoms like intrusive thoughts, panic attacks, and emotional numbness.
- **Cognitive Functioning:** Chronic stress can affect cognitive functions such as memory, concentration, and decision-making. Persistent stress can impair our capacity to focus, problem solve, and make informed decisions, affecting our performance at work, school, and in everyday life.

Recognizing the Signs and Symptoms of Burnout

Prolonged stress and excessive demands can lead to emotional, bodily, and mental weariness. Burnout is defined by emotions of extreme exhaustion, cynicism or detachment, and a diminished sense of accomplishment or effectiveness. Common signs and symptoms of burnout are:

1. **Exhaustion:** Exhaustion is defined as feeling physically and emotionally weary after having had a full night's rest. Burnout can leave you feeling

fatigued, empty, and unable to replenish your batteries, regardless of how much sleep you receive.

2. **Cynicism and Detachment:** Having a cynical or negative attitude towards work, relationships, or life in general. Burnout can cause emotions of detachment, indifference, and apathy, prompting you to retreat from activities or relationships that previously brought you joy or fulfillment.

3. **Reduced Performance:** A decrease in performance, productivity, and effectiveness at work, in relationships, or other aspects of life. Burnout can hinder your capacity to focus, problem-solve, and meet deadlines, resulting in lower performance and happiness.

4. **Emotional Distress:** Being stressed, anxious, or depressed as a result of burnout. Burnout can cause you to feel stressed, impatient, or emotionally numb, making it difficult to deal with daily obstacles and maintain strong relationships.

5. **Physical Symptoms:** Physical symptoms caused by persistent stress and burnout include headaches, muscle tension, sleep disruptions, and gastrointestinal issues. These physical symptoms can increase feelings of weariness and add to overall discomfort and anxiety.

Practical Strategies for Stress Management and Avoiding Burnout

1. **Prioritise self-care:** Make self-care a priority in your daily routine by including activities that encourage relaxation, renewal, and well-being. Schedule time for activities you enjoy, such as exercise, hobbies, meditation, or time with loved ones, and make rest a priority to replenish your batteries.

2. **Set boundaries:** Set clear boundaries between work and personal life to avoid burnout and maintain a good balance. Set work-hour boundaries, avoid taking on more duties than you can handle, and learn to say no to unreasonable demands or requests.

3. **Practice stress management techniques:** Deep breathing, progressive muscle relaxation, mindfulness meditation, and guided imagery are all stress-reduction and relaxation strategies that you can learn and practice.

These tactics can help you remain grounded, focused, and resilient in the face of adversity.

4. **Seek Support:** During stressful or burnout moments, seek support and encouragement from friends, family members, or trustworthy colleagues. Talking to someone you trust can provide perspective, validation, and emotional support, allowing you to better negotiate challenging situations.

5. **Delegate Tasks:** Delegate duties and responsibilities whenever possible to minimize your burden and alleviate feelings of overwhelm. Delegate duties that are outside of your area of expertise or that can be done more efficiently by others, allowing you to concentrate on priorities and areas where you can have the greatest influence.

6. **Practice Time Management:** Prioritise work, set realistic goals, and break down huge projects into smaller, more manageable pieces. To keep organized and focused, employ time management tactics such as to-do lists, calendars, and scheduling software. Avoid procrastination and overcommitting oneself.

7. **Cultivate Positive Relationships:** Make positive connections with coworkers, friends, and family members who offer encouragement, support, and camaraderie. Building strong social relationships can help mitigate the negative impacts of stress and burnout by instilling a sense of belonging and community.

8. **Take Breaks and Rest Periods:** Take regular pauses and rest intervals throughout the day to replenish your batteries and avoid burnout. Include short breaks in your workday to stretch, walk, or relax, and prioritize restful activities during evenings and weekends to encourage physical and mental regeneration.

Incorporating Hobbies and Activities for Joy

Hobbies and activities are occupations or pastimes that we do for enjoyment, relaxation, or personal fulfillment. They can take many forms, including creative endeavors like painting, writing, or crafting, physical activities like hiking, gardening, or sports, intellectual pursuits like reading, learning a new language, or solving puzzles, and social activities like volunteering, joining clubs or groups, or spending time with friends and family.

The Value of Hobbies and Activities for Well-Being

1. **Stress Reduction:** Hobbies and pastimes give a healthy release for stress and tension, helping us to unwind, relax, and recharge our batteries. Hobbies provide a respite from the stresses of daily life, lowering cortisol levels, encouraging relaxation, and improving general mood and well-being.

2. **Sense of Purpose:** Hobbies and pastimes provide us with a feeling of purpose and meaning by allowing us to explore our interests, learn new skills, and express ourselves creatively. Engaging in activities that are in line with our passions and values can provide us with a sense of fulfillment and happiness, as well as improve our general sense of purpose and well-being.

3. **Mental Stimulation:** Hobbies and pastimes excite the mind and improve cognitive performance, keeping our minds active and engaged. Hobbies, whether they involve solving puzzles, learning a new skill, or indulging in artistic pursuits, stimulate our minds, improve problem-solving abilities, and promote lifelong learning and growth.

4. **Social Connection:** Hobbies and pastimes provide for social connection and interaction, which fosters connections and builds community. Hobbies, whether they involve joining a club or group, engaging in team sports, or attending social events, give a common framework for connecting with others, developing friendships, and cultivating a sense of belonging and camaraderie.

5. **Emotional Well-Being:** Hobbies and activities can improve our emotional well-being by increasing feelings of enjoyment, fulfillment, and self-esteem. Hobbies provide an opportunity for self-expression and creativity, allowing us to pursue our interests, express our feelings, and develop a sense of self-worth.

Benefits of Integrating Hobbies and Activities

1. **Stress Relief:** Hobbies and pastimes provide a welcome relief from the demands of daily life, reducing tension, encouraging relaxation, and improving general mood and well-being. Hobbies, whether they involve immersing yourself in a creative project, losing yourself in a good book, or participating in outdoor activities, provide much-needed relief from the stresses of work, school, or other commitments.

2. **Enhanced Creativity:** Hobbies and pastimes foster creativity and invention, giving people a place to express themselves and explore their imagination. Painting, writing, and crafts allow us to express ourselves creatively, experiment with new ideas, and unleash our artistic skills.

3. **Improved Mental Health:** According to research, participating in hobbies and activities can improve mental health by lowering symptoms of anxiety, despair, and stress. Hobbies provide people with a sense of purpose and accomplishment, which increases self-esteem and promotes emotional well-being. In addition, hobbies provide a healthy coping mechanism for controlling negative emotions and increasing resilience in the face of adversity.

4. **Increased Physical Activity:** Many hobbies and pastimes need physical movement and exercise, which benefits physical health and fitness. Physical activities, such as hiking, gardening, dancing, or sports, can improve cardiovascular health, strengthen muscles and bones, and increase general physical fitness.

5. **Sense of Fulfilment:** Hobbies and activities that connect with our interests and passions can give us a sense of accomplishment and happiness. Hobbies, whether it's learning a new skill, completing a difficult project, or reaching a personal goal, provide possibilities for growth, achievement, and self-discovery.

Practical Strategies for Integrating Hobbies and Activities into Your Lifestyle

1. **Identify your interests:** Begin by recognizing your interests, passions, and hobbies, which bring you joy and fulfillment. Consider pastimes you enjoyed as a youngster, hobbies you've always wanted to try, or new interests you wish to pursue. Make a list of potential hobbies and activities that resonate with you and are consistent with your beliefs and priorities.

2. **Scheduled Time:** Make time for hobbies and interests by planning them into your daily or weekly schedule. Set out time in your calendar to pursue your hobbies, just like you would for work, appointments, or other obligations. Treat your interests as non-negotiable and prioritize them just like any other critical activity.

3. **Start Small:** Incorporate hobbies and interests into your life in reasonable amounts. Begin with activities that require little time, resources, or commitment, then progressively extend your repertory as you gain comfort and confidence. Remember that even tiny amounts of leisure time can have a huge impact on your well-being.

4. **Be flexible:** Be adaptable and open-minded about your hobbies and pastimes, allowing yourself to discover new interests and experiment with diverse endeavors. Don't be hesitant to venture outside of your comfort zone and attempt something new, even if it seems foreign or difficult at first. Accept the chance for development and discovery that comes with attempting new things.

5. **Set goals:** Set goals for your interests and activities to help you stay organized, motivated, and focused. Establish particular goals or milestones that you wish to reach, such as learning a new skill, completing a project, or engaging in a specific activity. Setting objectives can help you stay focused and involved, giving you a sense of purpose and achievement.

6. **Create a dedicated space:** Make a separate area in your home or setting for pursuing your hobbies and interests. Having a dedicated area for your hobbies, whether it's a cozy reading nook, a crafting corner, or a

home gym, may help foster involvement while also providing a sense of ownership and belonging.

7. **Prioritise Self-Care:** Make self-care a part of your hobby routine to ensure that you look after your physical, emotional, and mental health. Exercise, relaxation techniques, and mindfulness meditation are all examples of self-care activities that can help you recharge and maintain balance in your life.

8. **Share your interests:** Join clubs, groups, or communities of people who share your interests and hobbies. Participating in social activities relating to your hobbies can allow you to connect, collaborate, and bond with others, increasing your overall experience and building lasting relationships.

7

Chapter Six: Cognitive and Behavioral Techniques

Identifying and Challenging Negative Thoughts

Our thoughts have a significant impact on our emotions, behaviors, and general health. Negative thoughts, in particular, can be pervasive and harmful, causing emotions of anxiety, sadness, and self-doubt. However, by learning to recognize and fight negative beliefs, we can develop a more optimistic and resilient mentality that supports mental and emotional well-being.

Understanding negative thoughts

Negative thoughts are thought patterns that include pessimism, self-criticism, and an emphasis on perceived flaws, failures, or deficiencies. These ideas frequently occur spontaneously in reaction to stressful situations, eliciting feelings of melancholy, anxiety, or inadequacy. Common sorts of negative thoughts are:

1. **Catastrophizing:** Catastrophizing entails viewing circumstances in

the worst possible light and imagining the most disastrous outcomes. Catastrophizing entails exaggerating possible threats or hazards while underestimating one's ability to manage or overcome obstacles.

2. **All-or-Nothing Thinking:** Seeing problems in black and white, with no in-betweens or shades of grey. All-or-nothing thinking refers to extreme thought patterns, such as believing that everything is either wonderful or a complete failure, with no opportunity for nuance or compromise.

3. **Overgeneralization:** Overgeneralization is the process of drawing broad, sweeping conclusions from inadequate evidence or isolated instances. Overgeneralization occurs when bad experiences are extrapolated to all aspects of life, resulting in a distorted picture of reality and a sense of pessimism or despair.

4. **Personalization:** Accepting blame for events or consequences beyond one's control and attributing them to personal defects or shortcomings. Personalization is internalizing external events and blaming oneself for unpleasant consequences, even if they are unrelated to one's actions or behavior.

5. **Mind Reading:** Assuming we know what others are thinking or feeling without sufficient evidence, and attributing negative intentions or motives to their behavior. Mind reading entails forming erroneous assumptions about other people's thoughts, feelings, or intentions, which can result in misunderstandings and disputes.

Impact of Negative Thoughts

Negative thoughts can significantly affect our mental health, emotional well-being, and overall quality of life. If left unchecked, they can lead to:

- **Anxiety and Stress:** Negative thoughts fuel anxiety and stress, activating the body's stress response and increasing symptoms including racing thoughts, muscle tension, and difficulty concentrating. Chronic stress can cause a wide range of physical and mental health issues, including cardiovascular disease, digestive diseases, and mood disorders.

- **Depression:** Depression is characterized by negative thoughts, which contribute to emotions of hopelessness, worthlessness, and despair. Persistent negative thought patterns can feed a cycle of depression, resulting in retreat from social activities, diminished motivation, and impaired everyday functioning.
- **Low Self-Esteem:** Negative ideas lower self-esteem and self-worth, causing feelings of inadequacy, self-doubt, and self-criticism. Chronic self-criticism can undermine confidence, reduce resilience, and impede personal growth and development.
- **Relationship Problems:** Negative ideas can strain relationships and impede communication, resulting in disagreements, misunderstandings, and resentment. Unresolved negative ideas and emotions can block intimacy and connection, leading to feelings of loneliness and isolation.
- **Reduced Quality of Life:** Negative thoughts lower the overall quality of life by reducing opportunities for joy, fulfillment, and personal progress. Pervasive negative thinking patterns can skew our vision of reality, providing a flawed lens through which we see ourselves, others, and the world around us.

Identifying Negative Thoughts

Identifying negative beliefs is the first step in questioning and reframing them. Here are some ways to identify negative thought patterns:

- **Mindfulness:** Practice mindfulness to become more aware of your thoughts, feelings, and bodily sensations in the present moment. Pay attention to the content and tone of your thoughts without passing judgment, noting when unpleasant thoughts come and how they affect your mood and behavior.
- **Thought Records:** Maintain a thinking diary or journal to document your ideas and detect recurring patterns or topics. Record unpleasant thoughts as they arise, including the scenario or trigger that prompted them, the feelings they evoke, and any related physical sensations or behaviors.

- **Cognitive Distortions:** Become acquainted with typical cognitive distortions, such as catastrophizing, all-or-nothing thinking, and mind reading, and learn to identify them in your thinking. Recognize when these distortions arise in your thoughts and counter them with evidence-based reasoning.
- **Emotional Responses:** Pay attention to your emotional reactions to situations or occurrences, since they may reveal underlying negative ideas. Observe when you feel nervous, unhappy, or angry, and investigate any thoughts or beliefs that may be contributing to these feelings.
- **Physical Symptoms:** Pay attention to your body's physical feelings, which may indicate the presence of bad ideas or emotions. When you encounter symptoms like tension, headaches, or stomachaches, think about how they could be related to underlying negative thoughts or stressors.

Challenging negative thoughts

Once you've discovered your negative thoughts, question and reframe them to encourage a more optimistic and balanced outlook. Here are some ways to challenge negative thoughts:

- **Reality Testing:** Examine the data supporting and refuting your negative beliefs, using logic and reason to determine their accuracy and legitimacy. Ask yourself, "What evidence supports this thought?" and "Is there any evidence against it?"
- **Alternative Explanations:** Consider different explanations or interpretations for the situation or incident that caused the negative thought. Encourage yourself to produce alternative viewpoints and reframe the situation in a more balanced or positive way.
- **Best and worst-case scenarios:** Consider the best- and worst-case scenarios for the circumstance, weighing the probability and effects of each. Challenge catastrophic thinking by realistically examining prospective consequences and proposing more balanced alternatives.
- **Coping statements:** Create coping statements or affirmations to combat

negative thoughts and increase resilience. Make positive, encouraging phrases that challenge self-criticism and boost self-esteem, like "I am capable and competent" or "I am worthy of love and acceptance."

- **Cognitive Restructuring:** Use cognitive restructuring approaches to confront and change unfavorable thought patterns. Identify the underlying beliefs or assumptions that are causing negative thoughts and challenge them with evidence-based reasoning and different perspectives.
- **Reframing:** Negative ideas can be reframed by seeking silver linings or possibilities for growth and learning. Change your attention from what went wrong to what you can take away from the event, emphasizing resilience, resourcefulness, and personal development.
- **Gratitude Practice:** Cultivate gratitude as a counterpoint to negative thought patterns by concentrating on the good things in your life and what you are grateful for. Maintain a gratitude notebook, show appreciation to others, and savor moments of joy and beauty.
- **Self-Compassion:** Use self-compassion to reduce self-criticism and promote self-acceptance and kindness. Treat yourself with the same kindness and understanding that you would extend to a friend, accepting your flaws and shortcomings without passing judgment or condemnation.

Practicing Self-Compassion and Acceptance

Dr. Kristin Neff, a psychologist, invented the notion of self-compassion, which is based on mindfulness and self-kindness. It has three main components:

1. **Self-Kindness:** Being patient and understanding with oneself during times of sorrow or struggle, rather than severely criticizing or judging oneself. Self-kindness entails treating oneself with the same warmth, care, and support that one would extend to a friend in need.
2. **Common Humanity:** Recognising that suffering and imperfection are common experiences shared by all humans, rather than feeling alone or alone in our difficulties. Understanding that we are not alone in our struggles might help us feel more connected and compassionate towards

ourselves and others.

3. **Mindfulness:** Mindfulness entails approaching our experiences with mindfulness and nonjudgmental awareness rather than being overwhelmed by negative ideas or emotions. Mindfulness entails watching our thoughts and feelings with inquiry and compassion, allowing them to arise and pass without engaging in self-criticism or rumination.

Self-acceptance, on the other hand, is embracing oneself completely, including our qualities, shortcomings, triumphs, and failings. It means acknowledging and respecting our innate worth and value as humans, regardless of outward accomplishments or affirmation from others. Self-acceptance includes:

1. **Radical Self-Acceptance:** Accepting ourselves exactly as we are, without attempting to modify or improve ourselves to meet external norms or expectations. Radical self-acceptance entails lovingly identifying and appreciating our characteristics, idiosyncrasies, and flaws.

2. **Unconditional Self-Love:** Developing a strong love and appreciation for oneself, regardless of perceived imperfections or shortcomings. Unconditional self-love entails cultivating a positive and supportive connection with oneself, founded on self-respect, self-compassion, and self-care.

3. **Authenticity:** Accepting authenticity and vulnerability by being genuine to oneself, rather than hiding behind masks or personalities to impress others. Authentic self-acceptance is accepting our true selves, including our strengths, faults, and vulnerabilities, and living by our values and beliefs.

Benefits of Self-Compassion and Acceptance

1. **Improved Mental Health:** Studies have found that practicing self-compassion and acceptance leads to fewer symptoms of depression, anxiety, and stress. Cultivating a caring and accepting attitude towards

oneself enhances emotional resilience, self-regulation, and general psychological health.

2. **Increased Resilience:** Self-compassion and acceptance improve resilience by acting as a buffer against negative experiences and disappointments. When we treat ourselves with love and understanding, we can recover more easily and gracefully from obstacles, setbacks, and disappointments.

3. **Enhanced Self-Esteem:** Self-compassion and acceptance provide a positive feeling of self-worth and self-esteem. When we accept ourselves completely, flaws and all, we develop a strong sense of inner worth and confidence that is not dependent on outward validation or approval.

4. **Greater Empathy and Connection:** Self-compassion and acceptance build empathy and connection with others by instilling a feeling of shared humanity. When we recognize our common humanity and embrace our challenges and flaws, we are better able to empathize with others' experiences and form deeper bonds in our relationships.

5. **Reduced Self-criticism:** Self-compassion and acceptance. Reduce self-criticism and negative self-talk by providing a nicer, more compassionate alternative. When we respond to our mistakes and faults with compassion and understanding, we are less inclined to judge and criticize ourselves harshly.

Practical Strategies for Self-Compassion and Acceptance

- **Cultivate Self-Kindness:** Speak to oneself with gently, warmth, and support, especially during times of adversity or suffering. Offer yourself words of comfort and reassurance, just as you would to a close friend in need.
- **Embrace Imperfection:** Accept your defects and limits as natural parts of being human, rather than flaws to be rectified or corrected. Recognize that imperfection is a natural aspect of the human experience and that you are deserving of love and acceptance just the way you are.
- **Practice Mindfulness:** Develop mindfulness by paying nonjudgmental

attention to your thoughts, feelings, and bodily sensations in the present. When negative thoughts or feelings arise, notice them with inquiry and compassion, allowing them to pass without engaging in self-criticism or rumination.

- **Challenge Negative Self-Talk:** Question the truth and correctness of your critical ideas and views. Replace self-critical remarks with more balanced and sympathetic self-talk that emphasizes your talents, successes, and intrinsic value.

- **Set boundaries:** Set appropriate boundaries with yourself and others to safeguard your health and respect your needs and values. Practice saying no to unrealistic demands or expectations, and make self-care and self-compassion a priority in your daily life.

- **Practice Self-Care:** Prioritise self-care activities that nourish your body, mind, and soul, such as exercise, a healthy diet, enough sleep, relaxation techniques, and hobbies that make you happy and fulfilled.

- **Practice gratitude:** Cultivate gratitude by focusing on the positive elements of your life and expressing gratitude for the benefits, large and small, that you get every day. Keep a thankfulness notebook or simply spend a moment every day to focus on what you are thankful for.

- **Seek Support:** Seek support and encouragement from friends, family, or a therapist while you work towards self-compassion and acceptance. Surround yourself with people who support and validate you, and look for tools and communities that encourage self-compassion and well-being.

Behavior Activation and Goal Setting

Behavior activation is a treatment method based on behavioral psychology and cognitive-behavioral therapy (CBT). It focuses on recognizing and changing behavioral patterns that cause distress or impairment, to foster positive changes in mood, motivation, and functioning. Behavior activation is based on the idea that engaging in meaningful and rewarding activities can reduce depressive symptoms, boost motivation, and improve general well-being.

The key principles of behavior activation are

- **Activity Monitoring:** Begin by keeping track of your everyday activities and routines to detect patterns of behavior that may be causing you to feel distressed or depressed. Keep account of your activities, including the amount of time spent on each, the level of happiness or satisfaction felt, and any accompanying thoughts or emotions.

- **Activity arranging:** Once you've found patterns of behavior, start arranging activities that reflect your beliefs, interests, and ambitions. Break down projects into manageable chunks and include them in your daily or weekly routine, focusing on activities that produce a sense of accomplishment, enjoyment, or mastery.

- **Behavioral Activation:** Actively participate in planned activities, even if you don't feel like it or are faced with difficulties or challenges. Focus on taking tiny, regular actions toward your goals to gain momentum and confidence over time. To keep motivation and momentum going, use behavioral activation approaches including self-monitoring, problem-solving, and reinforcement.

- **Gradual Exposure:** Gradually expose oneself to activities or circumstances that you may have avoided out of fear, anxiety, or discomfort. Begin with small, controllable actions that progressively grow in difficulty or exposure over time. By confronting your anxieties and avoidance behaviors, you can develop resilience and confidence in your capacity to deal with situations.

Benefits of Behavioural Activation

1. **Improved Mood:** Engaging in meaningful and gratifying activities can help reduce depression symptoms while also boosting mood and general well-being. Behavior activation enhances positive emotions by focusing on tasks that provide joy, fulfillment, and a sense of accomplishment while decreasing feelings of despair, lethargy, and hopelessness.

2. **Increased Motivation:** Behaviour activation boosts motivation and

energy by instilling a sense of purpose, direction, and control. Setting goals and engaging in activities that correspond with your beliefs and interests can boost intrinsic motivation and keep you on track to meet your objectives.

3. **Enhanced Functioning:** Engaging in intentional and goal-directed activities boosts cognitive functioning, focus, and productivity. By breaking down tasks into small parts and arranging them into your daily routine, behavior activation improves efficiency, effectiveness, and general functioning in everyday life.

4. **Greater pleasure:** Behaviour activation fosters a sense of pleasure and fulfillment by encouraging participation in activities that are personally meaningful and fulfilling. Prioritizing activities that are consistent with your beliefs, interests, and goals can help you feel more purposeful, accomplished, and satisfied with your life.

Understanding Goal Setting

Goal setting involves creating specific, measurable, attainable, relevant, and time-bound (SMART) objectives to achieve within a specified timeframe. Goals, whether short or long-term, provide guidance, focus, and incentive for personal development and achievement. Setting clear and actionable goals fosters accountability, development, and overall success.

The key principles of goal setting are:

- **Specificity:** Set precise, explicit goals that outline exactly what you hope to accomplish. Clearly explain the desired objective, including what, when, where, and how you plan to achieve it. Avoid vague or confusing goals in favor of concrete and measurable objectives.
- **Measurability:** Create measurable criteria for tracking progress and success towards your objectives. Define particular measurements or indications that will help you track your progress and assess whether you are getting closer to your goal. Measurable goals set a clear standard

for measuring success and staying on track.

- **Achievability:** Set reasonable and attainable goals based on your current resources, abilities, and circumstances. Consider probable barriers or hurdles and develop solutions to overcome them. Choose goals that will stretch your abilities and challenge you to grow while remaining realistic.
- **Relevance:** Make sure your goals are consistent with your values, interests, and priorities. Select goals that are personally significant and relevant to your overall goals and ambitions. Aligning your goals with your beliefs boosts motivation and commitment, increasing the likelihood that you will remain focused and involved in achieving them.
- **Time-bound:** Set a specific timetable or deadline for attaining your objectives to create a sense of urgency and accountability. Break down major goals into smaller, more manageable actions with clear deadlines or milestones. Setting time-bound goals keeps you focused, motivated, and on pace to meet your objectives.

Benefits of Goal Setting

1. **Increased motivation:** Setting clear and achievable goals boosts motivation and commitment by giving people a sense of purpose, direction, and accountability. Goals provide you with something to aspire for and a purpose to be focused and disciplined in your efforts.
2. **Enhanced Focus and Clarity:** Goal planning improves concentration and clarity by outlining explicit objectives and priorities. Identifying your goals and breaking them down into concrete actions can help you stay organized, efficient, and effective in achieving them.
3. **Improved Performance:** Setting goals improves performance by establishing a framework for planning, activity, and evaluation. Goals provide a road map for success, guiding your efforts and keeping you on track to achieve your intended results.
4. **Greater Resilience:** Goal planning promotes resilience by instilling a growth mentality and a willingness to persevere in the face of adversity. Setting tough but attainable objectives and learning from failures or

losses will help you develop the resilience and perseverance required to overcome adversity and achieve success.

Effective Strategies for Behaviour Activation and Goal Setting

- **Identify values and priorities:** Begin by defining your beliefs, interests, and priorities to help guide your goal-planning process. Consider what is most important to you and what you hope to achieve in several aspects of your life, such as employment, relationships, health, and personal growth.
- **Set SMART goals:** Create SMART goals that are specific, measurable, attainable, relevant, and time-constrained. Break down larger goals into smaller, more manageable segments, and set explicit success and progress metrics. Write down your goals and revisit them regularly to keep focused and inspired.
- **Develop an Action Plan:** Create an action plan describing the measures you must take to achieve your goals. Divide chores into digestible parts and include them in your daily or weekly agenda. Set deadlines or milestones to hold yourself accountable and monitor your progress over time.
- **Prioritise Activities:** Choose activities that are consistent with your aims and values, focusing on tasks that will bring you closer to your intended outcomes. Identify activities that provide you joy, fulfillment, and a sense of accomplishment, and set aside time and energy to do them regularly.
- **Monitor Progress:** Regularly document your progress towards your goals, noting accomplishments, setbacks, and opportunities for growth. Review your goals and action plan regularly, making adjustments as appropriate to reflect changing circumstances or priorities.
- **Celebrate Achievements:** Celebrate your victories and milestones along the way, no matter how minor or trivial they may appear. Recognize your progress and achievements, and reward yourself for your hard work, persistence, and dedication.
- **Stay fluid and Adaptive:** Maintain a fluid and adaptive attitude to goal setting and behavior activation, altering your methods and tactics as needed to overcome hurdles or challenges. Accept the process of development

and learning, and be willing to pivot or change direction as needed.

Developing Healthy Coping Mechanisms

Coping mechanisms are the tactics, behaviors, or techniques that people use to manage stress, traverse challenging emotions, and deal with adversity. Coping methods can be adaptive or maladaptive, depending on how effective they are in promoting well-being and resilience. Adaptive coping methods encourage healthy emotional regulation, problem-solving, and resilience, whereas maladaptive coping mechanisms provide short comfort but eventually worsen stress and contribute to long-term emotional misery.

Key coping methods include:

1. **Problem-Focused Coping:** Problem-focused coping entails actively addressing the source of stress or hardship via problem-solving, planning, and action. This approach emphasizes finding practical answers to problems and making proactive efforts to change or improve the situation.

2. **Emotion-Focused Coping:** Emotion-focused coping is the process of controlling emotions and managing stress through relaxation, self-care, and emotional expression. This method emphasizes accepting and processing uncomfortable emotions rather than attempting to change external situations.

3. **Seeking Social Support:** Seeking social support is contacting friends, family members, or other trustworthy people for emotional, practical, or instrumental assistance. Social support fosters a sense of connection, belonging, and validation, allowing people to feel less alone in their challenges and more resilient in the face of hardship.

4. **Cognitive Restructuring:** Cognitive restructuring entails recognizing and confronting undesirable or maladaptive thoughts and beliefs that cause stress and emotional pain. This method emphasizes reframing negative thinking patterns and replacing them with more optimistic,

realistic, and adaptive perspectives.

5. **Acceptance and mindfulness:** Acceptance and mindfulness entail building present-moment awareness while embracing challenging ideas, feelings, and sensations without judgment or resistance. This technique focuses on nonjudgmental observation, self-compassion, and radical acceptance of one's own internal experiences.

Benefits of Healthy Coping Mechanisms

- **Enhanced Resilience:** Developing healthy coping mechanisms increases resilience by providing individuals with the skills and techniques they need to successfully handle life's obstacles and setbacks. Adaptive coping mechanisms encourage emotional flexibility, problem-solving abilities, and coping skills, allowing people to recover from adversity and thrive in the face of change.
- **Improved Mental Health:** Healthy coping mechanisms improve mental and emotional well-being by lowering stress, anxiety, and depression. Adaptive coping strategies assist individuals in regulating their emotions, managing stress more successfully, and cultivating a sense of inner peace and balance.
- **Better Relationships:** Healthy coping techniques promote efficient communication, conflict resolution, and emotional control, resulting in happier and more meaningful relationships. Individuals with adaptive coping skills are more capable of expressing their needs, setting limits, and maintaining healthy boundaries in their relationships.
- **Increased Productivity and Performance:** Healthy coping techniques boost productivity and performance by reducing distractions, improving focus, and improving cognitive function. Individuals who can effectively manage stress and emotions are better able to concentrate, solve problems, and perform at their best in a variety of settings, including work, school, and personal endeavors.
- **Greater Life Satisfaction:** Developing good coping skills increases life satisfaction and general well-being by instilling a sense of empowerment,

self-efficacy, and self-care. Individuals with adaptive coping skills are better able to face life's problems, follow their goals and objectives, and live a satisfying and meaningful life.

Practical Strategies to Develop Healthy Coping Mechanisms

- **Identify triggers:** Begin by identifying the precise stresses, triggers, or situations that cause intense emotional reactions or distress. Pay attention to the ideas, emotions, and physical sensations that occur in reaction to these triggers, and look for any patterns or repeated themes.
- **Develop Self-Awareness:** Practice self-awareness by monitoring your thoughts, feelings, and behaviors without passing judgment or criticism. Consider how you generally respond to stress and adversity, and become aware of any maladaptive coping techniques or behavioral patterns that may be contributing to emotional suffering.
- **Experiment with Coping tactics:** Try several coping tactics to see what works best for you in different situations. Test out a variety of adaptive coping mechanisms, including relaxation techniques, mindfulness practices, problem-solving skills, and social support networks, to find which ones work best for you.
- **Practice Self-Care:** Make self-care activities that nourish your body, mind, and soul a regular part of your routine. Make time for things that bring you joy, relaxation, and fulfillment, such as exercise, hobbies, creative outlets, and spending time with loved ones. Set limits and prioritize your well-being, even when faced with life's expectations and duties.
- **Cultivate Social Support:** Establish and maintain supportive relationships with friends, family members, and other trusted individuals who can provide emotional, practical, or instrumental assistance when required. Reach out to people for advice, encouragement, and insight, and be willing to help in return.
- **Develop resilience skills:** Increase your resilience by learning skills and tactics for adaptability, flexibility, and tenacity in the face of adversity. Practice reframing negative thought patterns, fostering gratitude,

creating realistic goals, and retaining a sense of humor in difficult circumstances.

- **Seek expert Help:** If you're having trouble coping with stress, worry, or other emotional issues, don't be afraid to seek help from a therapist, counsellor, or mental health expert. Professional help can give you extra resources, advice, and strategies for stress management and resilience.

8

Chapter Seven: Building Resilience and Emotional Strength

Cultivating Gratitude and Positivity

In a world full of obstacles, uncertainties, and setbacks, cultivating thankfulness and positivity is a transforming practice that may enrich our lives, nourish our souls, and foster a greater sense of well-being and fulfillment. Gratitude and positivity are more than ephemeral sentiments; they are strong attitudes and perspectives that may change our brains, lift our spirits, and improve our entire quality of life.

Understanding gratitude and positivity

Gratitude is the discipline of acknowledging and appreciating the blessings in our lives, large and small, that provide us joy, fulfilment, and significance. It entails recognizing the positive in our lives, expressing gratitude for the people, experiences, and opportunities that we come across, and creating a sense of abundance and satisfaction. Positivity, on the other hand, is the practice of maintaining an optimistic attitude toward life, focusing on the positive aspects of situations, and embracing the possibility of growth, resilience, and happiness.

Key principles of cultivating gratitude and positivity include:

1. **Mindfulness:** The cultivation of gratitude and positivity begins with mindfulness, often known as present-moment awareness. Mindfulness is the practice of paying attention to the present moment with openness, curiosity, and nonjudgment, allowing us to fully enjoy the beauty and richness of life as it unfolds around us.

2. **Perspective-adjusting:** Cultivating appreciation and positivity frequently entails adjusting our mindset from one of limitation or lack to one of abundance and possibilities. Instead of focusing on what we don't have or what's wrong, we can teach ourselves to see and appreciate the multitude of blessings and possibilities that surround us every day.

3. **Practice of Presence:** The practice of presence, or being fully involved and absorbed in the present moment, fosters gratitude and happiness. By focusing on the sights, sounds, and sensations of the present moment, we can feel tremendous amazement, wonder, and thankfulness for life's basic pleasures.

4. **Attitude of Appreciation:** Cultivating gratitude and optimism entails developing an attitude of appreciation and thankfulness for the blessings and gifts we have received. A magnificent sunset, a kind gesture from a friend, or a moment of laughter with loved ones are all opportunities for thanks and appreciation.

Benefits of cultivating gratitude and positivity

1. **Improved Mental Health:** Practicing thankfulness and positivity is linked to a variety of mental health benefits, including fewer symptoms of sadness, anxiety, and stress. Gratitude practices increase emotional resilience, pleasant mood, and overall psychological well-being.

2. **Enhanced Physical Health:** Gratitude and positivity have been related to better physical health outcomes, such as better sleep, less inflammation,

and stronger immune function. Adopting a grateful and optimistic attitude toward life might improve overall health and vitality.

3. **Increased Resilience:** Practicing appreciation and positivity helps people cope more effectively with hardship and disappointments. Individuals can recover more easily and gracefully from challenges by focusing on the positive parts of life and adopting a cheerful outlook.

4. **Stronger Relationships:** Gratitude and positivity improve relationships by encouraging deeper connections, trust, and closeness with others. Expressing gratitude and appreciation to loved ones deepens ties and sets off a positive feedback cycle of friendliness and reciprocity.

5. **Greater Life happiness:** Cultivating appreciation and optimism increases life happiness and well-being by instilling a sense of fulfillment, purpose, and meaning. Grateful people tend to have better levels of life satisfaction and subjective happiness, regardless of their circumstances.

Practical Strategies for Increasing Gratitude and Positivity

- **Keep a Gratitude diary:** Begin a daily or weekly gratitude diary in which you list three things you are grateful for every day. Think about the people, experiences, and benefits that offer you happiness, fulfillment, and gratitude. Writing down your blessings might help you feel more grateful and positive.

- **Mindful Appreciation:** Practice mindful appreciation by savoring the current moment and thoroughly immersing yourself in the sights, sounds, and sensations around you. Notice the beauty and richness of life all around you, and show gratitude for the little pleasures of everyday existence.

- **Express Gratitude to Others:** Take the time to recognize and appreciate the people in your life who make a difference, whether through a heartfelt thank-you note, a kind gesture, or a genuine statement of gratitude. Recognizing others' contributions develops connections and fosters a culture of appreciation.

- **Focus on the Positive:** Practice focusing on the positive qualities of a situation, even when faced with hurdles or difficulties. Find silver linings, opportunities for growth, and moments of beauty and grace amid life's ups and downs. Positively reframing unfavorable experiences might help you develop resilience and optimism.

- **Acts of compassion:** Show compassion and generosity to others as a way to express gratitude and share happiness. Acts of kindness, whether they involve volunteering your time, lending a helping hand, or expressing sympathy to someone in need, benefit both the recipient and the giver.
- **Positive Self-Talk:** Cultivate a positive inner conversation by using positive self-talk and affirmations. Replace self-critical thoughts with words of encouragement, compassion, and gratitude. Celebrate your skills, accomplishments, and distinguishing characteristics, and treat yourself with care and respect.
- **Surround Yourself with Positivity:** Surround yourself with people, places, and experiences that encourage and inspire you. Look for good influences, such as helpful friends, inspiring mentors, and uplifting media content, to promote gratitude, happiness, and optimism.

Finding Meaning and Purpose in Life

Meaning is the significance, value, or sense of purpose that people get from their experiences, relationships, and endeavors. It entails a strong sense of connectedness, coherence, and purpose in one's life, as well as congruence with one's values, beliefs, and goals. In contrast, the term "purpose" refers to the ultimate objective, goal, or direction that directs and gives meaning to one's life. It requires a feeling of purpose, direction, and dedication to a greater cause or calling.

The key elements of meaning and purpose are:

1. **Sense of Significance:** Feeling that one's life is meaningful entails a sense of significance, effect, or contribution to society. It comprises , the value and worth of one's existence, as well as the good impact one may

have on others and the world around them.

2. **Alignment with Values:** Finding meaning and purpose frequently entails matching one's behaviors, choices, and aspirations to firmly held values, beliefs, and principles. Living according to one's principles promotes a sense of integrity, authenticity, and congruence in one's life.

3. **Connection to Something Greater:** Meaning and purpose frequently involve a sense of connection to something more than oneself, whether it be a higher power, spirituality, a common cause, or the interconnection of all living beings. Feeling part of a bigger whole promotes a sense of belonging, purpose, and interconnectedness.

4. **Personal Growth and Fulfilment:** Finding meaning and purpose in life requires a dedication to personal development, self-discovery, and self-actualization. It requires getting out of one's comfort zone, accepting challenges and opportunities for progress, and constantly changing and expanding one's potential.

Benefits of Discovering Meaning and Purpose

1. **Enhanced Well-Being:** Studies have indicated that those who have a strong sense of meaning and purpose in life have better levels of subjective well-being, life satisfaction, and overall happiness. A feeling of purpose offers motivation, resilience, and fulfillment in the face of hardship.

2. **Improved Mental Health:** Finding meaning and purpose in life has been linked to a variety of mental health advantages, including lower levels of sadness, anxiety, and stress. A feeling of purpose encourages emotional resilience, self-efficacy, and a stronger sense of meaning and coherence in one's life.

3. **Increased Resilience:** Having a strong sense of meaning and purpose in life boosts resilience by giving a source of inner strength, inspiration, and perspective in the face of adversity. Individuals with a sense of purpose are better equipped to deal with obstacles, disappointments, and uncertainty, and they recover from adversity more easily and gracefully.

4. **Greater Sense of Fulfilment:** Pursuing meaning and purpose in life results in a greater sense of fulfillment, satisfaction, and contentment. Living by one's values, passions, and goals generates a profound sense of fulfillment and purpose that is independent of external circumstances or accomplishments.

5. **Improved Physical Health:** Research indicates that people who express a high sense of meaning and purpose in life have superior physical health results, such as lower rates of chronic disease, faster recovery from sickness, and a longer life expectancy. Having a sense of purpose encourages health-promoting behaviors like regular exercise, a nutritious diet, and stress management, which all contribute to overall well-being.

Practical Strategies for Discovering Meaning and Purpose

- **Reflect on Values and Beliefs:** Take some time to consider the essential values, beliefs, and principles that guide your life. Consider what is most important to you, what you are passionate about, and what gives your life meaning and purpose. Write down your values and beliefs, then consider how they influence your decisions and behaviors.

- **Identify Your Strengths and Passions:** Determine the skills, talents, and interests that provide you joy, fulfilment, and a sense of accomplishment. Consider the activities, hobbies, and pursuits that energize and inspire you, and figure out how to incorporate them into your life more fully.

- **Set Meaningful Goals:** Determine meaningful, purpose-driven goals that are consistent with your values, passions, and aspirations. Consider both short- and long-term goals that will challenge and excite you while also contributing to your sense of purpose and fulfillment. Break down major goals into smaller, attainable stages and devise a plan to achieve them.

- **Cultivate Connection and Contribution:** Make connections with others and contribute to something larger than yourself, whether via acts of kindness, volunteering, or community service. Engage in activities that allow you to positively impact others while also contributing to the well-being of your community and society.

- **Practice Gratitude and Mindfulness:** Cultivate gratitude and mindfulness to enhance your feeling of meaning and purpose in life. Take time each day to enjoy the benefits, opportunities, and experiences that enrich your life, and practice being aware of the beauty and richness of life as it unfolds around you.
- **Embrace Challenges and progress:** View challenges and possibilities for progress as a means of discovering meaning and purpose in life. Setbacks, failures, and challenges should be viewed as chances for learning, resilience, and personal growth, not as insurmountable impediments to success.
- **Seek Mentorship and advice:** Seek mentorship and advice from mentors, coaches, or trustworthy individuals who can provide insight, encouragement, and assistance on your path to discovering meaning and purpose. Surround yourself with people who inspire, elevate, and support your dreams and goals.

Developing Resilience to Life's Challenges

Resilience is the ability to tolerate, adapt to, and recover from adversity, trauma, or major life pressures. It entails using inner resources, coping abilities, and support networks to get through unpleasant situations and emerge stronger and more empowered on the other side. Resilience is not a fixed characteristic; rather, it is a dynamic process that may be developed and improved over time with deliberate effort, practice, and contemplation.

Key components of resilience include

1. **Adaptability:** Resilience entails being adaptable and flexible in the face of change, uncertainty, and adversity. It means viewing adversities as chances for growth, learning, and personal development rather than impassable barriers.
2. **Emotional Regulation:** Resilience is the ability to effectively regulate and manage emotions in the face of stress, adversity, and uncertainty.

It comprises adopting good coping methods, such as mindfulness, relaxation techniques, and positive self-talk, to navigate unpleasant emotions while maintaining inner calm and stability.

3. **Problem-Solving Skills:** Resilience is defined as the ability to identify and successfully solve issues or impediments through problem-solving skills, critical thinking, and resourcefulness. It means confronting problems with optimism, ingenuity, and tenacity, and looking for answers rather than succumbing to despair or helplessness.

4. **Social Support:** Resilience entails accessing and utilizing social support networks, which include friends, family members, mentors, and community resources, to provide emotional, practical, and instrumental assistance during times of need. It requires developing connections and relationships that promote and sustain resilience in the face of adversity.

Benefits of Developing Resilience

- **Improved Mental Health:** Developing resilience can lead to improved mental health, such as reduced anxiety, depression, and PTSD symptoms. Resilient individuals are better able to cope with stress, hardship, and trauma, as well as have a good attitude toward life even when confronted with problems.
- **Increased Emotional Well-Being:** Resilient people tend to have higher levels of emotional well-being, such as increased happiness, life satisfaction, and general psychological health. They are better prepared to deal with life's ups and downs with grace, resilience, and a sense of inner calm and balance.
- **Enhanced Coping abilities:** Developing resilience improves coping abilities and techniques for dealing with stress, adversity, and uncertainty. Resilient people have a repertoire of adaptive coping techniques, such as problem-solving, emotional regulation, and seeking social support, which allow them to effectively traverse tough situations and recover from setbacks.
- **Greater Sense of Purpose:** Building resilience promotes a stronger sense

of purpose, meaning, and direction in life. Even in the face of tragedy, resilient people can discover meaning and value in their experiences, as well as preserve a feeling of hope, optimism, and purposeful involvement with life.

- **Improved ties:** Resilient people have stronger, more supportive ties with their friends, family, and community networks. They are better equipped to form and sustain strong, meaningful relationships that provide emotional, practical, and instrumental assistance in times of need.

Practical Strategies to Develop Resilience

1. **Cultivate Self-Awareness:** Start with establishing self-awareness and recognizing your talents, shortcomings, and opportunities for improvement. Reflect on your past experiences with resilience and adversity, and identify the coping processes, tactics, and resources that helped you get through challenging times.

2. **Foster strong Relationships:** Invest in developing and strengthening strong relationships with friends, family members, mentors, and other supportive people who can offer emotional, practical, and instrumental assistance when needed. Seek out possibilities for connection, communication, and collaboration to promote resilience and well-being.

3. **Develop Coping Skills:** Learn and practice ways for effectively managing stress, hardship, and uncertainty. Explore practices like mindfulness, relaxation, deep breathing, and positive self-talk to improve emotional control and resilience in the face of adversity.

4. **Set Realistic Goals:** Set reasonable, attainable goals that are consistent with your values, interests, and aspirations. Break down major goals into smaller, more doable tasks, and develop a strategy for attaining them over time. Celebrate your progress and victories along the way, and change your goals to reflect new circumstances or priorities.

5. **Cultivate Optimism:** Develop a sense of optimism and hope in the face of hardship. Practice reframing negative thought patterns and

concentrating on the positive side of things, even when faced with difficulties or setbacks. Encourage gratitude, appreciation, and resilience in the face of life's ups and downs.

6. **Embrace challenges as opportunities:** Accept obstacles and disappointments as opportunities for personal growth, learning, and development. Approach obstacles with a curious, open, and resilient mindset, and look for possibilities for self-reflection, adaptation, and progress amid adversity.

7. **Seek Support and Guidance:** Don't be afraid to seek help and advice from others when necessary. Reach out to friends, family members, mentors, or mental health experts for advice, support, and resources to help you negotiate difficult situations and develop resilience.

Embracing Change and Adaptability

Change is the process of transitioning or transforming from one state, condition, or circumstance into another. It can manifest in a variety of ways, including changes in relationships, jobs, health, or surroundings, and can be both external and internal. In contrast, adaptability refers to the ability to change, evolve, and thrive in the face of changing situations, settings, or expectations. It requires adaptability, resilience, and an openness to new experiences, ideas, and perspectives.

The key factors of change and adaptability are

1. **Acceptance:** Acceptance is the first step towards embracing change; it acknowledges that change is an unavoidable and natural element of life. Instead of opposing or denying change, create an open, curious, and accepting attitude toward new experiences, opportunities, and possibilities.

2. **Flexibility:** Adaptability refers to the ability to adjust and respond effectively to changing situations, difficulties, and opportunities. It means letting go of rigidity and instead embracing flexibility, inventiveness,

and creative problem-solving in the face of uncertainty.

3. **Resilience:** Developing resilience is critical for handling change with ease and confidence. Resilience entails recovering from failures, obstacles, and adversity while also finding strength, meaning, and purpose in challenging situations. It requires developing inner resources, coping skills, and support networks to face life's ups and downs with resilience and drive.

4. **Growth Mindset:** Embracing change necessitates adopting a growth mindset, which holds that our abilities, talents, and intelligence can be developed through effort, practice, and education. It comprises seeing difficulties and setbacks as chances for growth, learning, and self-improvement, rather than as insurmountable hurdles or failures.

Benefits of Accepting Change and Adaptability

- **Personal Growth and Development:** Accepting change encourages personal growth and development by pushing us to leave our comfort zones, explore new possibilities, and push our limits. It allows for self-discovery, learning, and self-improvement while also encouraging resilience, adaptation, and creativity in the face of uncertainty.

- **Increased Resilience and Well-Being:** Developing adaptability boosts resilience and well-being by providing us with the tools and resources we need to face life's challenges confidently and gracefully. It encourages emotional control, problem-solving, and efficient coping techniques while also instilling a sense of inner strength, confidence, and self-efficacy.

- **Enhanced Problem-Solving Skills:** Accepting change encourages the development of competent problem-solving, critical thinking, and decision-making abilities. It inspires us to approach issues with curiosity, creativity, and ingenuity, as well as to look for new solutions to challenging problems.

- **Improved Relationships and Communication:** Embracing change encourages empathy, understanding, and flexibility in our dealings with others. It motivates us to actively listen, speak openly, and work effectively with others, even when our thoughts or ideas disagree.

Practical Strategies for Accepting Change and Developing Adaptability

- **Cultivate Mindfulness:** Mindfulness can help you develop awareness, presence, and acceptance of your current situation. Mindfulness meditation, deep breathing exercises, or body scan techniques can help you create inner peace, clarity, and resilience amid change and uncertainty.
- **Practice Flexibility:** Practice flexibility by seeing uncertainty, ambiguity, and change as opportunities for growth and learning. Let go of the demand for control or assurance, and instead accept life's fluidity and unpredictability with curiosity, openness, and flexibility.
- **Develop Resilience Skills:** Learn resilience skills and coping mechanisms so you can navigate change with confidence and resilience. Create a toolkit of adaptive coping methods, such as problem-solving, emotion management, and social support, to help you negotiate life's problems with resilience and determination.
- **Set Realistic Goals:** Set realistic goals. Set reasonable, attainable goals that are consistent with your values, aspirations, and priorities. Break down major goals into smaller, actionable actions and develop a strategy for accomplishing them over time. Be flexible and adaptive in your approach, adapting your goals and techniques as needed to reflect changing circumstances or priorities.
- **Seek Support and Guidance:** Ask friends, family members, mentors, or mental health experts for advice, encouragement, and resources to help you negotiate change and foster adaptability. Reach out to others for assistance and be willing to provide it in return.
- **Embrace the Growth Mindset:** View challenges and setbacks as chances for growth, learning, and self-improvement. Approach change with curiosity, optimism, and a readiness to learn from experience, and see mistakes or failures as significant chances for personal growth and discovery.

9

Chapter Eight: Seeking Professional Help and Treatment Options

Therapy Options for Depression

Depression is a complicated mental health issue that affects millions of individuals worldwide. While medicine may be necessary for some people, therapy is also important for controlling and conquering depression. Therapy provides a safe and supportive atmosphere in which people can explore their ideas, emotions, and behaviors, build coping mechanisms, and gain insight into the root reasons for their sadness.

Treatment Options for Depression

1. Cognitive-Behavioral Therapy (CBT): Cognitive-behavioral Therapy (CBT) is a highly researched and successful treatment for depression. CBT focuses on recognizing and addressing negative thought patterns and beliefs that contribute to depression, as well as learning coping skills and behavioral techniques to help manage symptoms. Individuals in CBT learn to recognize and reframe erroneous thought patterns, build problem-solving abilities, and gradually engage in activities that provide pleasure or satisfaction.

2. Interpersonal psychotherapy (IPT): Interpersonal therapy (IPT) is a time-limited treatment that aims to improve interpersonal interactions and address interpersonal issues that lead to depression. IPT aims to assist individuals in identifying and resolving interpersonal issues, improving communication skills, and developing stronger connections with others. IPT usually focuses on four major areas: grieving and loss, role changes, interpersonal conflicts, and interpersonal deficiencies.

3. Psychodynamic Therapy: Psychodynamic Therapy examines how past experiences, emotions, and unconscious processes impact current behavior and relationships. Psychodynamic treatment seeks to identify underlying tensions and unresolved issues that lead to depression, frequently by looking at childhood events, interpersonal patterns, and defense mechanisms. Individuals can obtain a better knowledge of their ideas, feelings, and behaviors by practicing insight and self-awareness, as well as working towards resolution and healing.

4. Acceptance and Commitment Therapy (ACT): Acceptance and Commitment Therapy (ACT) is a mindfulness-based therapy that emphasizes accepting and embracing challenging ideas and feelings, rather than attempting to modify or avoid them. ACT strives to assist individuals in clarifying their beliefs, setting meaningful goals, and taking determined action towards living a full life, especially in the face of depression or other problems. ACT emphasizes awareness, acceptance of inner experiences, and the significance of taking values-based action.

5. Dialectical Behavior Therapy (DBT): Dialectical Behaviour Therapy (DBT) was initially created for borderline personality disorder but has now been adapted to treat depression and other mood disorders. DBT combines cognitive-behavioral techniques with mindfulness skills to help individuals regulate emotions, tolerate distress, improve interpersonal relationships, and develop effective coping strategies. DBT typically consists of individual therapy, group skill training, phone coaching, and consultation team meetings.

6. Mindfulness-based cognitive therapy (MBCT): Mindfulness-based cognitive therapy (MBCT) is a combination of cognitive therapy and mindfulness techniques designed to avoid relapse in people who have had recurrent depression. MBCT teaches people how to build present-moment awareness and acceptance of painful thoughts and feelings, as well as how to break free from automatic rumination and negative thinking patterns that can lead to relapse. Individuals who include mindfulness practices in their daily lives can create a more sympathetic and nonjudgmental attitude towards their circumstances, lowering the likelihood of depression relapse.

7. Behavioral Activation: Behavioral activation therapy involves engaging in rewarding activities to reduce depression. Behavioral activation seeks to identify and change tendencies of avoidance and withdrawal that contribute to depression, as well as to enhance engagement in activities that provide a sense of pleasure, success, and mastery. Behavioral activation assists people in leading more full and meaningful lives by focusing on boosting positive reinforcement and decreasing negative reinforcement.

Choosing the Right Treatment

When contemplating depression therapy choices, it is critical to select a method that is tailored to your tastes, requirements, and goals. Here are some considerations to consider when selecting the appropriate therapy:

- **Treatment Preferences:** Consider your treatment preferences, such as the type of therapy approach, format (individual, group, or online), and number of sessions. Some people prefer structured, goal-oriented therapies like cognitive behavioral therapy or IPT, whereas others prefer more exploratory or insight-oriented techniques like psychodynamic therapy.
- **Therapist competence:** Look for a therapist with experience and competence in treating depression, as well as training in the specific therapeutic technique you want to pursue. Inquire about their credentials, training,

and experience working with depression patients, as well as their therapeutic approach and treatment philosophy.

- **Personal Compatibility:** Think about how well you and the therapist get along. A solid therapeutic alliance and a trustworthy, supportive relationship with your therapist are critical for positive treatment outcomes. Trust your intuition and find a therapist with whom you feel at ease, understood, and appreciated.
- **Treatment Goals:** Clarify your therapy goals and objectives, and share them honestly with your therapist. Whether you want to relieve symptoms, strengthen relationships, develop coping skills, or gain insight into underlying issues, it's critical to discuss your objectives and expectations with your therapist so that your therapy matches your needs and priorities.
- **Cost and Accessibility:** Think about the cost, accessibility, and practical aspects of therapy, such as insurance coverage, out-of-pocket fees, location, and scheduling options. When making a decision, research various therapy alternatives and providers in your area, taking into account variables such as convenience, affordability, and accessibility.

Medication and Psychiatric Treatment

Medication and psychiatric treatment refer to a variety of strategies used to manage and treat mental health illnesses such as depression, anxiety, bipolar disorder, schizophrenia, and others. Psychiatric treatment may include medication, psychotherapy, counseling, hospitalization, or a mix of these techniques, depending on the type and severity of the individual's symptoms and diagnosis.

Medication Options:

1. **Antidepressants:** Antidepressants are drugs that are widely used to treat depression, anxiety disorders, and other mood disorders. They function by raising neurotransmitter levels in the brain, including serotonin, norepinephrine, and dopamine, which are considered to regulate mood,

emotions, and stress response. Antidepressants are classified into four types: selective serotonin reuptake inhibitors (SSRIs), serotonin-norepinephrine reuptake inhibitors (SNRIs), tricyclic antidepressants (TCAs), and monoamine oxidase inhibitors.

2. **Anxiolytics:** Anxiolytics, often known as anti-anxiety drugs, are medications used to treat anxiety disorders, panic attacks, and other ailments. They function by modifying neurotransmitter activity in the brain, focusing on the gamma-aminobutyric acid (GABA) system, which regulates anxiety and stress responses. Common anxiolytics include benzodiazepines, buspirone, and beta-blockers.

3. **Mood Stabilizers:** Mood stabilizers are drugs that treat bipolar disorder and help to stabilize mood fluctuations, preventing or reducing the frequency and severity of manic and depressed episodes. They function by regulating neurotransmitter activity in the brain, specifically dopamine, serotonin, and glutamate. Common mood stabilizers include lithium, anticonvulsants (e.g., valproate, carbamazepine, lamotrigine), and atypical antipsychotics.

4. **Antipsychotics:** Antipsychotics, also known as neuroleptics, are drugs that treat psychotic diseases such as schizophrenia, bipolar disorder with psychotic symptoms, and severe mood disorders. They act by inhibiting dopamine receptors in the brain, which reduces the intensity of psychotic symptoms such as hallucinations, delusions, and disorganized thinking. Antipsychotics are classed as typical (first-generation) or atypical (second-generation) based on their mode of action and side effects.

5. **Stimulants:** Stimulants are drugs that treat attention-deficit/hyperactivity disorder (ADHD) and narcolepsy by raising dopamine and norepinephrine levels in the brain, which improves attention, focus, and impulse control. Methylphenidate (Ritalin, Concerta) and amphetamines (Adderall, Vyvanse) are two common forms of stimulants.

Considerations For Medication Use

While medicine can be quite useful in managing and treating mental health conditions, it is critical to approach medication use with caution and careful thought. Here are some crucial factors to consider when contemplating medication for mental health treatment:

- **Individualized Treatment:** Medication should be provided on an individual basis, taking into account the patient's diagnosis, symptoms, medical history, co-occurring conditions, and treatment preferences. What works for one person may not work for another, so consult with a skilled healthcare provider to determine the best prescription and dose for your specific needs.
- **Side Effects:** All drugs can cause side effects ranging from moderate to severe, which vary depending on the medication, dosage, and individual variables. Common adverse effects of psychiatric drugs include drowsiness, dizziness, nausea, weight gain, sexual dysfunction, dry mouth, and constipation. It is critical to address potential side effects with your healthcare professional and consider the advantages and dangers of pharmaceutical use.
- **Monitoring and Follow-up:** When taking psychiatric medications, it is critical to see your doctor regularly to assess treatment response, monitor for adverse effects, and alter medication dosage or regimen as needed. Attend all regular appointments, report any concerns or changes in symptoms to your healthcare practitioner, and follow their drug management recommendations.
- **Long-Term usage:** Some psychiatric drugs may be recommended for short-term usage to relieve acute symptoms, while others may be used as long-term maintenance therapy to avoid symptom recurrence or relapse. It is critical to discuss the intended duration of drug treatment with your healthcare provider and consider the potential advantages and hazards of long-term medication use.
- **Psychotherapy and Counselling:** Medication is frequently used in con-

junction with psychotherapy, counseling, or other non-pharmacological modalities to provide comprehensive mental health treatment. Therapy can help people build coping skills, increase self-awareness, and address underlying issues that contribute to their symptoms, thereby supplementing the benefits of medicine and facilitating long-term healing.

- **Lifestyle Factors:** In addition to medicine and therapy, food, exercise, sleep, stress management, and social support are important in managing and treating mental health conditions. Adopting good lifestyle practices can increase medication effectiveness, and general well-being, and lower the chance of symptom relapse or recurrence.

Exploring Alternative and Complementary Therapies

Alternative and complementary therapies are methods of health and healing that differ from traditional medical techniques. While some alternative therapies have been used for centuries in traditional healing systems such as Ayurveda, Traditional Chinese Medicine (TCM), and indigenous medicine, others have emerged in recent years as people seek non-pharmacological and integrative approaches to health and wellness.

Alternative and complementary therapies rely on the following key principles:

1. **Holistic Approach:** Alternative and complementary therapies approach wellness holistically, recognizing the individual as a whole person with mind, body, and spirit. Rather than treating only symptoms or specific health disorders, these therapies seek to restore balance, harmony, and vitality to all elements of the individual's existence.

2. **Individualized Care:** Alternative and complementary therapies emphasize individualized care, tailoring treatments and interventions to each person's specific needs, preferences, and circumstances. When establishing treatment plans, practitioners consider the patient's health history, lifestyle, beliefs, and goals.

3. **Integrative Medicine:** Integrative medicine is the practice of combining conventional medical treatments with alternative and complementary therapies to deliver comprehensive, patient-centered care. Integrative medicine aims to bridge the gap between traditional and alternative approaches to health and healing, recognizing the importance of both in promoting overall health and wellness.

4. **Self-Empowerment:** Alternative and complementary therapies enable people to take an active role in their health and well-being by giving them tools, techniques, and resources to help them heal and care for themselves. These therapies emphasize the importance of lifestyle variables like food, exercise, stress management, and social support in preserving health and avoiding illness.

Types of Alternative and Complementary Therapies

1. **Acupuncture:** Acupuncture is a vital component of Traditional Chinese Medicine (TCM) that includes inserting thin needles into particular spots on the body to stimulate energy flow, balance Qi (life energy), and promote healing. Acupuncture is used to treat a variety of ailments, including pain, stress, anxiety, digestive difficulties, and musculoskeletal issues.

2. **Herbal Medicine:** Herbal medicine, also known as botanical medicine or phytotherapy, is the use of plants and plant extracts to prevent, relieve, or treat a variety of medical diseases. Herbs are chosen for their therapeutic characteristics and are commonly utilized in the form of teas, tinctures, capsules, and topical applications. Ginseng, echinacea, valerian, chamomile, and turmeric are some of the most commonly used herbal medicines.

3. **Mind-Body Therapies:** Mind-body therapies are a broad category of techniques that focus on the relationship between the mind and body and its impact on health and well-being. Mind-body therapies include meditation, mindfulness, yoga, tai chi, qigong, biofeedback, guided imagery, hypnosis, and relaxation techniques. These activities encourage

relaxation, stress reduction, emotional balance, and self-awareness, which improves general health and well-being.

4. **Energy Healing:** Modalities such as Reiki, Healing Touch, and Therapeutic Touch use the body's subtle energy systems to promote healing, balance, and relaxation. Practitioners utilize light touch or non-contact techniques to direct universal life force energy (Qi, Prana, or Ki) to the recipient, thereby eliminating blockages, restoring energy flow, and assisting the body's natural healing processes.

5. **Chiropractic Care:** Chiropractic care focuses on the diagnosis and treatment of musculoskeletal problems, particularly those involving the spine and nervous system. Chiropractors employ manual adjustments, spinal manipulation, and other treatments to realign the spine, reduce pain, increase mobility, and promote general health and well-being.

6. **Massage Therapy:** Massage therapy is the manipulation of the body's soft tissues, such as muscles, tendons, ligaments, and connective tissue, to promote relaxation, relieve pain, increase circulation, and improve general well-being. Various massage techniques, including Swedish massage, deep tissue massage, sports massage, and aromatherapy massage, are utilized to address various health needs and preferences.

Benefits of Alternative and Complementary Therapies

Alternative and complementary therapies have numerous benefits for physical, emotional, mental, and spiritual health. Some of the primary benefits are:

1. **Pain Relief:** Acupuncture, massage therapy, and chiropractic care are examples of alternative therapies that can effectively treat acute and chronic pain disorders such as back pain, arthritis, headaches, and muscle tension.

2. **Stress Reduction:** Mind-body therapies, energy healing, and relaxation techniques are extremely successful at lowering stress, promoting relaxation, and restoring nervous system equilibrium. These techniques can help people deal with stress, anxiety, and other mental health issues,

boosting their general resilience and well-being.

3. **Improved Mental Health:** Alternative therapies such as meditation, mindfulness, yoga, and tai chi have been demonstrated to improve mood, alleviate depression and anxiety symptoms, and boost emotional well-being. These activities encourage self-awareness, emotional regulation, and resilience, allowing people to better cope with life's problems.

4. **Enhanced Immune Function:** Some alternative therapies, such as acupuncture, herbal medicine, and energy healing, are thought to boost immune function and the body's natural healing mechanisms. These therapies, which restore balance to the body's energy systems and promote optimal immune system function, can help avoid sickness and enhance overall health and vitality.

5. **Increased Self-Awareness:** Alternative therapies like meditation, mindfulness, and guided imagery encourage self-awareness, introspection, and self-discovery, allowing people to gain a better understanding of themselves, their emotions, and their deepest wishes and goals. These practices promote a sense of connection, purpose, and meaning in life, ultimately improving general well-being and quality of life.

Considerations for Alternative and Complementary Therapies

Alternative and complementary medicines have many potential benefits, but they should be approached with caution and discernment. Here are some important points to keep in mind when researching alternative therapies:

- **Evidence-Based Practice:** While many alternative therapies have been used for centuries and have anecdotal evidence to support their usefulness, not all of them have been extensively investigated or confirmed successfully through scientific research. When contemplating alternative health and wellness solutions, it is critical to look for evidence-based techniques and contact credible sources.
- **Safety and Regulations:** Some alternative therapies may provide hazards or adverse effects, especially if used poorly or by unqualified personnel.

Before beginning treatment, it is critical to conduct research on the safety and regulation of alternative therapies, including practitioner qualifications, training, and certification. Be aware of practitioners who make exaggerated claims or offer rapid fixes.

- **Integration with traditional Care:** Alternative therapies should supplement, not replace, traditional medical care. It is critical to inform your healthcare physician about any alternative therapies you are investigating and discuss how they may fit into your current treatment plan. Your healthcare practitioner can advise you on how to use alternative therapies safely and appropriately, as well as help you coordinate your care more efficiently.

- **Personal Choices and Values:** When deciding on alternative therapies, keep your health and wellness choices, values, and beliefs in mind. Explore various modalities and techniques to see what speaks to you and connects with your health and well-being objectives and priorities.

Understanding the Role of Support Groups

Support groups are meetings of people who come together to share their experiences, struggles, and successes connected to a particular issue or concern. These groups offer a supportive and nonjudgmental environment in which people may openly express themselves, receive acceptance and understanding from others, and gain practical guidance, encouragement, and coping skills.

The key qualities of support groups are:

1. **Shared Experience:** Support groups bring together people who have had the same experience, such as a medical condition, life event, or mental health issue. Whether it's cancer survivors, bereaved parents, or people suffering from depression, the common experience fosters a sense of community and understanding among group participants.
2. **Peer Support:** In support groups, people provide empathy, affirmation,

and encouragement to one another based on their own experiences and viewpoints. Peer support helps people feel understood, accepted, and appreciated, which fosters a sense of belonging and connection within the group.

3. **Emotional Validation:** Support groups allow people to express their thoughts, feelings, and emotions freely and without judgment. Sharing experiences with others who have been through a similar journey can help to affirm one's feelings and experiences, lessening feelings of loneliness, shame, and self-doubt.

4. **Information Sharing:** Support groups are an excellent source of information and resources for people facing similar issues. Group members can exchange practical suggestions, resources, and methods for dealing with their ailment or circumstance, as well as information about local therapies, services, and support networks.

5. **Empowerment and Advocacy:** Support groups encourage people to take an active role in their health and well-being by offering a forum for advocacy, education, and empowerment. Group members can advocate for their own needs, rights, and interests, as well as create awareness and encourage good change in their communities.

Types of Support Groups

Support groups can address a variety of challenges, concerns, and interests. Some common forms of support groups are:

1. **Condition-Specific Support Groups:** These groups bring together people who have the same medical condition or diagnosis, such as cancer, diabetes, chronic pain, or autoimmune illnesses. Condition-specific support groups allow people to share their stories, learn from others, and receive comfort and understanding from those who understand what they're going through.

2. **Bereavement Support Groups:** Bereavement support groups are intended to assist people cope with the loss of a loved one, whether via

death, divorce, or separation. These groups offer a safe and friendly environment in which people can process their grief, share memories, and find comfort and peace in the presence of others who are also mourning.

3. **Mental Health Support Groups:** These groups bring together people who are dealing with mental health issues like depression, anxiety, bipolar disorder, schizophrenia, or PTSD. These groups allow people to express their challenges, achievements, and coping skills while also receiving support, encouragement, and validation from others who understand their situation.

4. **Carer Support Groups:** These groups are intended to help people who are caring for a loved one with a chronic disease, disability, or aging-related issue. These groups allow carers to express their struggles, disappointments, and concerns while also receiving practical guidance, emotional support, and respite from their caregiving responsibilities.

5. **Parenting Support Groups:** Parenting support groups allow parents to share their experiences, struggles, and accomplishments when parenting children. These groups may focus on specific parenting topics such as breastfeeding, child development, special needs parenting, or single parenting, providing parents with a supportive community as well as resources and information.

Benefits of Support Groups

Support groups can provide several benefits to persons experiencing problems, crises, or transitions in their lives. Some of the primary benefits are:

- **Validation and Understanding:** Support groups offer a secure and validating environment in which people can communicate their thoughts, feelings, and experiences freely and without judgement. Sharing experiences with others who have been through a similar journey can help to affirm one's feelings and experiences, lessening feelings of loneliness, shame, and self-doubt.

- **Emotional Support:** Support groups provide emotional support and empathy from peers who understand the problems and struggles that people face. Group members can offer support, encouragement, and reassurance, as well as practical information and coping skills for dealing with challenging situations.

- **Sense of Belonging:** Support groups create a sense of belonging and connection among people who share a similar experience or issue. Finding solidarity and camaraderie inside the group can make people feel less alone, more understood, and accepted, increasing their sense of community and belonging.

- **Practical Advice and Resources:** Individuals facing similar issues can benefit from support groups, which provide vital information and resources. Group members can exchange practical suggestions, methods, and resources for dealing with their ailment or circumstance, as well as information about local therapies, services, and support networks.

- **Empowerment and Advocacy:** Support groups encourage people to take an active role in their health and well-being by offering a forum for advocacy, education, and empowerment. Group members can advocate for their own needs, rights, and interests, as well as create awareness and encourage good change in their communities.

Considerations for joining a support group

When considering joining a support group, it's important to keep the following factors in mind:

- **Group Dynamics:** Consider the dynamics and structure of the support group, such as its size, meeting frequency and format, and the group leader's facilitation style. Choose a group that makes you feel comfortable and supported, and where you can share openly and honestly.

- **Confidentiality and Privacy:** Ensure that the support group respects the confidentiality and privacy of the information shared among members. Trust and secrecy are vital for fostering a secure and supportive environment in which people can share their experiences and concerns.

- **Compatibility:** Determine whether the support group is a good fit for you in terms of emphasis, goals, and membership. Choose a group that meets your needs, interests, and ideals, and where you feel welcome and welcomed by the other members.

- **Professional Guidance:** Some support groups are conducted by qualified professionals such as therapists, counsellors, or social workers, and others are peer-led or self-help groups. Depending on your needs and interests, you may prefer a group directed by a professional or led by peers who have had comparable experiences.

- **Additional Support:** While support groups can be a great source of encouragement and support, they may not be enough to deal with complex or serious situations on their own. Consider whether you would benefit from extra help, such as individual therapy, counseling, or medical treatment, in addition to attending a support group.

10

Chapter Nine: Maintaining Progress and Preventing Relapse

Strategies for Long-Term Recovery

S tarting the journey of recovery from addiction, mental illness, or any other significant life problem is a brave and transformational experience. While meeting short-term goals and milestones is crucial, the ultimate goal of recovery is to stay healthy and flourishing in the long run.

Understanding long-term recovery

Long-term recovery is a path of continuous growth, healing, and transformation that lasts beyond the initial stages of recovery. It entails establishing new behaviors, beliefs, and habits that promote health and well-being, as well as developing resilience, self-awareness, and self-compassion. Long-term recovery is more than just refraining from substances or managing symptoms; it is about living a life full of purpose, meaning, and connection.

The key concepts of long-term recovery are:

1. **Commitment to Change:** Long-term recovery necessitates a dedication to change and progress, as well as a willingness to face challenges, setbacks, and hurdles along the path. It entails recognizing the need for change, establishing goals and aspirations for the future, and taking regular action to effect positive change in one's life.

2. **Holistic Approach:** Long-term rehabilitation includes a comprehensive approach to wellness, addressing the physical, emotional, mental, and spiritual dimensions of health and well-being. It entails nourishing all aspects of oneself, including physical health, mental health, relationships, employment, hobbies, and spirituality, to live a balanced and full life.

3. **Self-Awareness and Reflection:** Long-term rehabilitation entails learning self-awareness and reflection abilities, as well as investigating one's thoughts, feelings, beliefs, and behaviors. It is about identifying the underlying reasons and triggers of addiction, mental illness, and other difficulties, as well as adopting healthy coping and stress-response strategies.

4. **Support and Connection:** Long-term recovery relies on the understanding and support of others. It entails establishing a strong support network of friends, family, peers, mentors, therapists, and support groups that may offer encouragement, direction, and accountability along the journey.

5. **Lifelong Learning and Growth:** Long-term healing is an ongoing process of learning, growth, and personal development. It entails actively seeking out opportunities for education, skill development, and personal growth, as well as welcoming new experiences, challenges, and possibilities for self-discovery and expansion.

Strategies For Long-Term Recovery

- **Establishing Healthy Routines and Habits:** One of the most successful long-term rehabilitation strategies is to develop healthy daily routines and habits that promote health and well-being. This could include prioritizing proper sleep, exercise, diet, and self-care routines, as well as establishing boundaries, managing stress, and practicing mindfulness and relaxation techniques.

- **Building a Strong Support Network:** Long-term recovery requires a strong support network that includes friends, family, peers, mentors, therapists, and support groups. These people may offer encouragement, direction, and accountability, as well as practical and emotional support during difficult times.

- **Continuing Education and Skill-Building:** Long-term healing requires ongoing education, skill-building, and personal development activities. This could include pursuing formal education or vocational training, attending workshops or seminars, discovering new hobbies or interests, or looking for possibilities for personal development and self-improvement.

- **Practicing Self-Care and Stress Management:** Prioritizing self-care and stress management methods is critical for preserving balance and well-being during long-term recovery. This could include engaging in regular self-care activities like exercise, meditation, writing, or spending time outside, as well as learning effective stress management strategies like deep breathing, progressive muscle relaxation, or guided imagery.

- **Cultivating Meaningful Relationships:** Developing and maintaining meaningful relationships with others is critical for long-term rehabilitation. This could include repairing and strengthening existing relationships, as well as making new connections with supportive and understanding people who share similar values and interests.

- **Setting and Working Towards Goals:** Setting realistic and attainable future goals is critical for keeping motivation and momentum during long-term recovery. This may entail establishing short-term, medium-term, and long-term goals in numerous aspects of life, such as employment, education, relationships, health, and personal development, and then taking regular action to achieve them.

- **Practicing Mindfulness and Self-Compassion:** Mindfulness and self-compassion are essential for sustaining emotional balance and resilience in long-term recovery. This is being present in the moment, accepting oneself and one's experiences without judgment, and responding to oneself with kindness and understanding in tough situations.

- **Staying connected to recovery resources:** Staying linked to recovery tools and support networks is critical for retaining accountability and motivation in long-term rehabilitation. This may entail attending monthly support group meetings, therapy sessions, or alumni activities, as well as staying current on breakthroughs in addiction treatment and recovery.

- **Embracing a Sense of Purpose and Meaning:** Finding and accepting a sense of purpose and meaning in life is critical to long-term rehabilitation. This might include defining one's values, passions, and strengths, as well as developing meaningful objectives and participating in activities that bring joy, fulfillment, and a feeling of purpose.

- **Celebrating Milestones and Progress:** Celebrating milestones and success along the road to recovery is critical for preserving motivation and morale. Whether it's commemorating a period of sobriety, completing a personal goal, or conquering a huge struggle, taking the time to acknowledge and celebrate one's accomplishments can increase confidence, self-esteem, and drive to keep going forward.

Recognizing Early Warning Signs

Early warning signals are subtle indications or symptoms that occur before the onset or worsening of a condition or issue. These indications can take many forms, including physical, emotional, behavioral, cognitive, and interpersonal indicators. While early warning indicators vary depending on the ailment or challenge, they frequently contain common characteristics, such as changes in mood, behavior, or functioning that deviate from an individual's norm.

Early warning indications have the following key characteristics:

1. **Subtlety:** Early warning indicators are frequently subtle and may go overlooked or dismissed as trivial by the person experiencing them or those around them. These indications may be subtle changes in mood, behavior, or functioning that emerge gradually over time and do not immediately raise red flags.

2. **Variability:** Early warning symptoms can vary in severity, duration, and frequency from person to person, as well as over time. While some people see clear and regular warning signs, others may have more subtle or intermittent clues that appear and disappear unexpectedly.

3. **Contextualization:** Early warning indicators should be recognized in light of the individual's specific circumstances, experiences, and background. Past trauma, current stresses, environmental triggers, and social support networks all have an impact on how early warning indicators emerge and are interpreted.

4. **Individualized Response:** Effectively responding to early warning indicators necessitates an individualized strategy that takes into consideration the person's unique needs, preferences, and circumstances. What works for one person may not work for another, making it critical to adjust interventions and support measures to the individual's specific situation.

Common Early Warning Signs

While early warning signs differ depending on the ailment or issue, some similar symptoms may indicate the need for additional evaluation or intervention. It's crucial to remember that having one or more of these symptoms does not always indicate a specific diagnosis, but it may demand further investigation and evaluation by a knowledgeable practitioner. Some common early warning indicators are:

1. Changes in mood or emotion:

- *Persistent sadness, hopelessness, or despair*
- *Irritability, agitation, or mood swings*
- *Loss of interest or pleasure in previously enjoyed activities*
- *Feelings of guilt, worthlessness, or self-blame*
- *Increased anxiety, worry, or tension*
- *Suicidal thoughts, ideation, or self-harming behaviors*

2. Changes in behavior or functioning:

- *Increased or decreased energy levels.*
- *Changes in appetite, weight, or eating habits*
- *Sleep disturbances, including insomnia and hypersomnia.*
- *Difficulty focusing, making judgments, or remembering*
- *Withdrawing from social activities, interests, or relationships*
- *Engaging in dangerous or reckless behavior*

3. Changes in Physical Health:

- *Consistent bodily complaints, such as headaches, stomachaches, or exhaustion*
- *Changes in appetite, weight, or eating habits*
- *Digestive problems, such as nausea, vomiting, or diarrhea*
- *Unexpected aches, pains, or discomfort*
- *Changes in sleep habits, such as trouble falling or staying asleep*
- *Enhanced vulnerability to sickness or illnesses*

4. Changes in Cognitive Function:

- *Difficulty concentrating, focusing, or paying attention*
- *Memory problems or forgetfulness*
- *Confusion, disorientation, or cognitive impairment*
- *Racing thoughts or difficulty organizing thoughts*
- *Impaired decision-making or problem-solving abilities*

· *Slowed thinking or speech patterns*

5. Changes in interpersonal relationships:

· *Increased conflicts or arguments with family members, friends, or colleagues*
· *Withdrawal from social interactions or avoidance of social situations*
· *Difficulty communicating or expressing oneself effectively*
· *Changes in relationship dynamics, such as increased dependency or clinginess*
· *Loss of interest in maintaining relationships or participating in social activities*
· *Feeling disconnected or alienated from others*

Responding to Early Warning Signs

To effectively respond to early warning signs, take a proactive and holistic approach that addresses the underlying causes and triggers of symptoms. It is critical to take early warning symptoms seriously and seek appropriate assistance, support, and resources as soon as possible. Here are some ideas for responding to the early warning symptoms.

· **Self-awareness and self-monitoring:** Develop self-awareness and self-monitoring skills to detect changes in mood, behavior, or function as they occur. Pay close attention to small signs and indications from your body, emotions, and thoughts, and keep track of any patterns or trends over time.
· **Seek Professional Evaluation and Assessment:** If you detect any persistent or alarming early warning symptoms, consult a trained healthcare physician, therapist, counsellor, or mental health professional. These experts can perform a thorough evaluation, examine your symptoms and concerns, and make an accurate diagnosis and therapy suggestions.
· **Develop coping strategies and self-care practices:** Create coping techniques and self-care activities to reduce stress, regulate emotions, and promote overall well-being. This could include practicing relaxation

techniques, mindfulness meditation, deep breathing exercises, or participating in things that provide joy and fulfillment.

- **Create a Support Network:** Create a support network of friends, family members, peers, mentors, and support groups that can offer encouragement, empathy, and practical assistance during difficult times. When you need support, validation, or guidance, reach out to trusted people.
- **Establish healthy habits and routines:** Establish healthy habits and routines that promote physical, emotional, and mental wellness. This could include prioritizing proper sleep, exercise, diet, and self-care routines, as well as setting boundaries, controlling stress, and using effective time management techniques.
- **Explore Treatment Options and Resources:** Investigate therapy choices and resources that can address your issues and requirements. Individual treatment, group therapy, medication, support groups, self-help literature, online resources, and alternative and complementary therapies are all possible options.
- **Communicate openly and honestly:** Open and honest communication with your healthcare providers, therapists, and support network about your symptoms, concerns, and needs is essential. Be proactive in getting help and advocating for yourself; don't be afraid to ask questions or communicate your treatment preferences and goals.
- **Monitor progress and adjust as needed:** Monitor your progress and make adjustments to your treatment plan as appropriate based on your reaction to interventions and changes in symptoms. Be willing to try new ways or adjust existing ones to better meet your needs and promote recovery and wellness.

Creating a Relapse Prevention Plan

Relapse is a typical and often stressful event in the recovery process, defined as the return to addictive behaviors, destructive patterns, or symptoms of mental illness following a time of abstinence or stability. Relapse can happen for a variety of reasons, including exposure to triggers, stress, emotional anguish, social pressure, or underlying psychiatric problems. While relapse can be upsetting and disheartening, it is critical to understand that it is a normal component of the recovery process and does not indicate failure or weakness. Instead, relapse allows for contemplation, learning, and growth, and it can act as a catalyst for reinforcing one's commitment to recovery.

The key components of a relapse prevention plan are:

1. **Self-Awareness and Monitoring:** Developing self-awareness and monitoring skills is critical for identifying early warning signals and causes of a relapse. Pay close attention to changes in mood, behavior, or thought patterns, as well as external influences including stressful events, social surroundings, or substance-related signs. Keep a notebook or log to record your thoughts, feelings, and behaviours, and look for patterns or trends that may suggest an increased risk of relapse.

2. **Identify Triggers and High-Risk Situations:** Identifying triggers and high-risk scenarios that may increase the possibility of relapse is an essential step in creating a relapse prevention strategy. Triggers can be internal, such as negative feelings, desires, or erroneous thinking habits, or external, such as people, places, or activities linked to substance abuse or harmful behavior. Stress, boredom, loneliness, negative emotions, social pressure, and exposure to addictive substances or cues are all common triggers.

3. **Coping Strategies and Skills:** Developing coping strategies and skills to manage triggers and high-risk situations is key to preventing relapse. Determine what healthy coping skills work for you, such as relaxation techniques, mindfulness meditation, exercise, hobbies, or social support networks. To increase resilience and lower the risk of relapse, practice coping techniques regularly and incorporate them into your daily routine.

4. **Lifestyle Changes and Self-Care Practices:** Making lifestyle modifications and prioritizing self-care routines that promote health and well-being is critical for sustaining stability and resilience during recovery. This may involve eating a well-balanced diet, exercising regularly,

prioritizing sleep, using stress-management skills, and participating in activities that offer joy and fulfillment. Pay attention to your physical, emotional, and spiritual needs, and prioritize self-care in your daily routine.

5. **Social Support and Accountability:** Having a robust support network, including friends, family, peers, mentors, therapists, and support groups, is crucial for preventing relapse and maintaining recovery. Surround yourself with people who understand and support your journey and can offer encouragement, counsel, and accountability during difficult times. Stay in touch with your support network and reach out for assistance when needed.

6. **Healthy Relationships and Boundaries:** Maintaining healthy connections and setting boundaries with others is crucial for ensuring recovery and well-being. Surround yourself with good people who understand and support your sobriety or recovery goals. Communicate freely and honestly with others about your needs, boundaries, and expectations, and be willing to enforce boundaries as needed to protect your sobriety and well-being.

7. **Relapse Response Plan:** A relapse response plan describes precise procedures to take in case of a relapse or recurrence of symptoms. This may entail reaching out to your support network for assistance, seeking professional help from a therapist or counselor, attending support group meetings, reevaluating your treatment plan, and implementing coping strategies and self-care practices to address the underlying triggers and challenges.

8. **Continual Evaluation and Adjustment:** Effective relapse prevention requires ongoing evaluation and adjustment based on progress, experiences, and changing requirements. Review your plan regularly, identify any areas for improvement or modification, and make changes as needed to keep it relevant, thorough, and in line with your recovery goals and priorities.

Developing an Individualised Relapse Prevention Plan

Assess your strengths, problems, triggers, and requirements to create a personalized strategy for recovery and wellness. Here are some methods to help you establish an individual relapse prevention plan:

1. **Self-assessment and Reflection:** Start by self-assessing and reflecting on your recovery journey, including past experiences, triggers, problems, strengths, and aspirations. Identify any patterns or trends in your substance use or addictive behaviours, as well as any risk factors for relapse.

2. **Identify the triggers and warning signs:** Identify your triggers and warning signals of relapse, such as stress, negative emotions, cravings, or exposure to substances or addiction-related cues. When identifying your triggers, be as thorough and detailed as possible, and take into account both internal and external situations that may contribute to relapse.

3. **Develop coping strategies and skills:** Create a repertoire of coping methods and abilities to efficiently handle triggers and high-risk circumstances. Consider both short-term coping skills for dealing with acute cravings or urges, as well as long-term tactics for treating root causes and strengthening resilience. Coping techniques should be practiced regularly and integrated into your daily routine to improve your capacity to deal with stress and temptation.

4. **Build a Support Network:** Create a supportive network of friends, family, peers, mentors, therapists, and support groups to guide you through your recovery journey. To avoid isolation and loneliness, reach out to trusted folks for assistance, guidance, and encouragement as required, and stay connected to your support network.

5. **Establish Healthy Habits and Routines:** Establish healthy habits and routines that support physical, emotional, and mental well-being. Examples include regular exercise, balanced nutrition, appropriate sleep, and stress management skills. Prioritise self-care methods that encourage relaxation, enjoyment, and fulfillment, and set aside time for things that

offer you joy and satisfaction.

6. **Create a Relapse Response Plan:** Create a relapse response plan outlining precise procedures to take in case of a relapse or recurrence of symptoms. This may entail reaching out to your support network for assistance, seeking professional help from a therapist or counselor, attending support group meetings, reevaluating your treatment plan, and implementing coping strategies and self-care practices to address the underlying triggers and challenges.

7. **Continuous Evaluation and Adjustment:** Evaluate and adapt your relapse prevention strategy regularly to reflect your progress, experiences, and changing requirements. Review your plan regularly, identify any areas for improvement or modification, and make changes as needed to keep it relevant, thorough, and in line with your recovery goals and priorities.

Building a Support Network for Ongoing Support

Support networks are critical in the recovery path because they provide individuals with the encouragement, direction, and accountability they need to face the challenges of recovery with strength and resilience. Whether you're recovering from addiction, mental illness, trauma, or other life issues, having a support network can help you stay motivated, stay on track with your treatment goals, and avoid relapse or symptom recurrence.

Key advantages of establishing a support network include:

- **Emotional Support:** A support network offers emotional support and validation, allowing people to communicate their thoughts, concerns, and challenges in a safe and supportive setting. Having someone listen, empathize, and offer support can make people feel understood, validated, and less alone in their challenges.
- **Practical aid:** A support network can provide clients with practical aid and resources to help them manage the practical problems of recovery, such as identifying treatment alternatives, obtaining healthcare services,

managing finances, or finding housing. Having someone to help with transportation, daycare, or meal preparation can make the recuperation process more bearable and less burdensome.

- **Accountability:** A support network holds you accountable and motivates you to stick to your treatment goals and recovery plans. Knowing that others are rooting for you and holding you accountable for your actions can boost your motivation, commitment, and persistence in achieving your recovery goals.

- **Role Modelling:** A support network can provide positive role models and examples of successful rehabilitation, instilling hope and optimism in people who are struggling. Seeing others who have conquered comparable obstacles and made significant progress can boost confidence, belief in oneself, and motivation to persevere in the face of adversity.

- **Social Connection:** A support network fosters social connection and a sense of belonging, allowing people to feel connected, respected, and included in a community of understanding and supporting peers. Building meaningful relationships with individuals who have faced similar experiences and struggles can help to lessen feelings of isolation, loneliness, and alienation while also promoting a sense of camaraderie and solidarity in recovery.

Elements of an Effective Support Network

Building an effective support network entails cultivating relationships with individuals who can offer support, direction, and encouragement during recovery. Here are some essential components of an effective support network:

- **Diverse Perspectives:** Look for people with diverse perspectives, backgrounds, and experiences who may provide unique insights, ideas, and perspectives on recovery. Having a diverse support network can help you widen your understanding, challenge your assumptions, and gain a more holistic view of recovery.

- **Trusted Relationships:** Build relationships with people you trust and feel comfortable talking to about your challenges, anxieties, and objectives. To build a strong support network, cultivate relationships based on mutual respect, honesty, and confidentiality.

- **Positive Influence:** Surround yourself with positive influencers who encourage and inspire you to be your best self. Avoid relationships with people who could jeopardize your recovery or divert you from your goals, and instead seek out those who genuinely support and believe in your potential to succeed.
- **Reciprocity:**Cultivate reciprocal relationships in which you and your support network share support, encouragement, and assistance. Provide support and encouragement to individuals in your network, and be open to receiving help and support when required.
- **limits:** Set clear limits in your relationships with others to safeguard your recovery and well-being. Be forceful in stating your needs, preferences, and limits, and be willing to enforce them if required to maintain your sobriety, health, and safety.
- **Accessibility:** Develop relationships with people who are readily available to offer support and assistance when needed. Whether it's through in-person interactions, phone conversations, text messages, or online communication, make sure you have several ways to engage with your support team.
- **Diversity of Support Systems:** Expand your support network by involving friends, family members, peers, mentors, therapists, support groups, and community organizations. A varied support network guarantees that you have access to a variety of services, resources, and viewpoints to match your changing requirements.

Strategies for Building a Support Network

Building a support network requires time, effort, and intentionality, but the advantages outweigh the hurdles. Here are some ideas for developing a strong support network to provide ongoing support and encouragement during recovery:

- **Reach Out to Friends and Family:** Begin by reaching out to friends and family members who are supportive and understanding of your rehabilitation process. Share your experiences, concerns, and aspirations with them, and ask for their help, encouragement, and support as you face the obstacles of recovery.

- **Join Support Groups:** Groups like Alcoholics Anonymous (AA), Narcotics Anonymous (NA), SMART Recovery, and peer-led support groups can provide vital peer support, encouragement, and guidance from people who have firsthand experience with addiction or mental illness. Attend meetings regularly, actively participate, and interact with other members to form meaningful connections and support.

- **Seek Professional Help:** Consult therapists, counsellors, or mental health professionals who specialize in addiction therapy or mental health rehabilitation. A competent expert can offer you personalized support, guidance, and treatment to help you address underlying issues, build coping skills, and maintain long-term recovery.

- **Participate in Community Activities:** Join community activities, volunteer work, or recreational groups that share your interests and values. Connecting with others through common activities and interests can lead to possibilities for socialization, friendship, and support outside of standard treatment settings.

- **Use Online Resources:** Take advantage of online resources, forums, and communities that offer support, knowledge, and resources to those in recovery. Websites, blogs, social media groups, and online forums can help you connect with others who have faced similar experiences and obstacles, as well as give a venue for sharing tales, seeking advice, and offering support.

- **Attend Workshops and Events:** Attend workshops, seminars, or events about addiction recovery, mental health, or personal development to meet people who share your aims and interests. These events allow you to learn, network, and form relationships with people who are dedicated to personal improvement and wellness.

- **Develop Peer Relationships:** Form relationships with people who are also in recovery or have conquered similar issues. Peer support can provide encouragement, affirmation, and inspiration, as well as practical advice and direction from individuals with firsthand experience with recovery.

- **Practice Active Listening and Empathy:** Practice active listening and empathy. In your contact with others, use active listening and empathy, and show real interest in their experiences, feelings, and perspectives. Demonstrate empathy, understanding, and compassion for others, and provide support and encouragement without passing judgment or condemnation.

- **Be upfront and Authentic:** When interacting with others, be upfront and honest about your personal experiences, problems, and triumphs. Authenticity develops true connections based on mutual understanding and shared experiences while also establishing trust and rapport with people.

- **Be Patient and Persistent:** Establishing a support network requires time, patience, and persistence, so be patient with yourself and others as you work through the process. Do not be discouraged by failures or rejections; instead, continue to reach out and connect with individuals who can help and encourage you on your recovery journey.

11

Conclusion

In concluding our exploration of depression in women, let's reflect on the key points we've uncovered throughout this journey. We've delved into the definition and gender differences of depression, debunked myths, and examined its profound impact on various aspects of women's lives. We've discussed practical strategies, mindfulness practices, and the importance of seeking help and building support systems.

To all our readers, I want to extend heartfelt encouragement and support. Dealing with depression can feel daunting, but you are not alone in this journey. Remember, there is strength in seeking help and reaching out for support. You have the power to navigate through the challenges and emerge stronger on the other side.

As we conclude, let's carry forward the knowledge, resilience, and empowerment gained from this exploration. Let's continue to prioritize our mental health, practice self-care, and support one another in our journey towards healing and well-being.

With warm regards and best wishes for your continued resilience and growth,

[MATHA J. RUSSELL]